RADIATION AND HEALTH

RADIATION
AND HEALTH

William Valentine Mayneord

ALDINETRANSACTION
A Division of Transaction Publishers
New Brunswick (U.S.A.) and London (U.K.)

First paperback printing 2012
Copyright © 1964 by The Nuffield Provincial Hospitals Trust.

This book is printed on acid-free paper that meets the American National Standard for Permanence of Paper for Printed Library Materials.

Library of Congress Catalog Number: 2011030267
ISBN 978-1-4128-4282-2
Printed in the United States of America

Library of Congress Cataloging-in-Publication Data

Mayneord, William Valentine.
    Radiation and health / William Valentine Mayneord.
        p. ; cm.
    Originally published by the Nuffield Provincial Hospitals Trust, 1964.
    Includes bibliographical references and index.
    ISBN 978-1-4128-4282-2 (alk. paper)
        I. Title. [DNLM: 1. Radiation Effects. 2. Radiation Protection. WN 650] LC classification not assigned

615.8'4--dc23

2011030267

CONTENTS

Radiation and Health

INTRODUCTION

In the first Rock Carling Monograph [1] Sir John Charles noted Bentham's use of the term 'mesology' and its related 'social mesology' as being the discipline concerned with the effects upon human beings as individuals or in society of temperature, light, humidity, gravity, atmospheric pressure, meteorology and electrical influences, food and drink, urbanization, sanitary conditions, occupation, domesticity, religion, institutions, laws and psychological factors.

My task, it seems, is to add 'ionizing radiation' to this formidable catalogue and so define the science of 'radiomesology', snatching the word from the mouths of those who concern themselves with the social consequences of the British Broadcasting Corporation. It is to be noted that Bertillon, who in 1873 rescued the term 'mesology' from oblivion, maintained that there are only two possible ways of modifying man either individually or in the mass. We must either modify his ancestry (clearly possible so far as future generations are concerned) or his natural and social environment.

This distinction neatly sketches the main divisions of radiomesology and even provides appropriate pigeonholes for natural and artificial radioactivity. We observe at once that the study of the effects of radiation on man is part of an immensely wider sociological survey. We guess that our study of radiation and health is likely to show close analogy with that of many other physical factors considered in the same context and is not lightly to be regarded as a thing *sui generis*. The number of ways in which a living organism can react to a stimulus is smaller than the variety of stimuli to which it may be exposed.

We are concerned with 'Radiation and Health' and doubtless a logical discussion would commence with a definition of both. By radiation we shall mean only 'ionizing radiation', rather reluctantly omitting sunlight and near visible radiation and confining ourselves to X and gamma rays, as well as corpuscular radiations of high energy such as alpha and beta particles and neutrons. All these entities convey energy to living tissues upon which they fall and in which they are absorbed, thus bringing about physical and chemical changes. These changes, often following complex metabolic paths, sometimes express themselves as biological alterations of medical significance. This, then, is the fundamental rôle of radiation in our context and radiation might be defined in these terms.

But who shall define 'Health'? Do we insist upon the perfect equilibrium and perfect harmony in the individual postulated by Galen and to be attained only in rare moments of life, or be content with a mere absence of clinically detected disease? Shall we take as our basic unit a complete human population, a whole man, a single somatic or germ cell, a chromosome or a gene? Many people now speak of 'Health' as a definable and measurable quantity, characteristically expressing it in a negative way via mortality or morbidity statistics of populations. Yet it is obvious that the patterns of life throughout the world vary so much that no single standard can be set for all peoples, nor even for the same people at different times. Moreover, health status has to be looked at from a community as well as from a personal point of view and social well-being may be regarded as a predisposing condition of individual health. In the search for quantitative criteria many 'health indicators' [2] have been suggested, often classified into three groups: (*a*) those associated with the health status of persons or populations in a given area, for example, vital statistics, proportional mortality ratio, life expectation, nutrition, infant mortality, deaths from communicable diseases, and many others; (*b*) those related to physical environmental conditions having a more or less direct bearing on the health status of the population in the area under review, for example percentage of the population receiving protected water supply; and (*c*) those concerned with health-service activities directed to improvement of health conditions, for example the availability and use of hospitals. From our point of view obviously none of these criteria is satisfactory, though the exercise may lead to the writing down of a statistic somehow related to 'Health'. Quantitative data concerning the effects of atomic energy and radiations on the well-being of a community are necessarily largely lacking, but this question of defining health, or rather selecting an arbitrary indicator of so-called health and trying to correlate it with radiation, is of fundamental importance to our subject. We may doubt with Alice 'whether you *can* make words mean so many different things', but like the scornful Humpty Dumpty we pay them extra and show which is Master. Nowadays we extend our patronage to numbers too and this perhaps is even more dangerous.

We have later attempted a balance of 'good' and 'bad' effects of radiation in our society and there is a great temptation to use impressive numerical data as valid criteria to justify our opinions, but it is well to remember the crudity of such concepts of health and well-being before becoming too enmeshed in them.

As a physicist I naturally believe that to be 'numerate' is as important as to be 'literate', but some years of experience in medical physics have taught me that part of the pleasurable impact of numerical data may arise from the power of a number to obscure uncomfortable uncertainty as to what we are talking about.

No subject has at once suffered or gained more from the glare of world publicity than the study of radiation and health. Insistent daily demands for immediate answers leave scientists little time for balanced judgements and well-informed replies, yet had public pressure not been so great, would resources for research and observation have been so profusely forthcoming? If we have sometimes been forced to appear more dogmatic and certain in our opinions than our scientific consciences approved of, at least we stood more chance of having the resources to improve those opinions. We have, too, suffered great changes in climate of opinion. Fifty years ago Radium was the wondrous substance leading to the elimination of disease, the discovery of the 'Essence of Life' and perhaps to a life of ease and happiness to all mankind. Today it is a dangerous substance, the least quantity of which is furtively contained in thick lead caskets and handled with the utmost caution. We must take account of such changing opinions, hoping to be forgiven if we adopt like the doctor described by Rock Carling[3] 'a mood of diffident scepticism which long experience of changing medical opinion and belief has taught us'. Remembering, too, with Lecky that the success of an opinion depends 'much less upon the force of its arguments, or upon the ability of its advocates, than upon the predisposition of society to receive it'.

Part I

The nature, origin and effects of radiation

Chapter 1

RADIATION AND THE METABOLISM
OF RADIOACTIVE MATERIALS

It may be useful to start with a short account of the physical nature of ionizing radiation and its interaction with the human body, though the story has often been told and we wish to avoid more technical detail than necessary.

The radiations of interest to us may be divided into two main groups, on the one hand electrically charged or uncharged particles (alpha and beta particles and neutrons), on the other electromagnetic radiations (X and gamma rays). Physical studies of the fundamental nature of radiation have blurred the outline of the distinction between them since the former may be thought of as energetic micro-projectiles in their own right, while the latter occur as discrete packets of energy (quanta) which on absorption give rise to similar secondary particles. We still await a formal unified concept of radiation, but from a biological point of view this is of little consequence. The important point is that all types of radiation transfer energy and cause alterations in all materials in which they are absorbed, including those of the biosphere. The particles of interest, such as alpha or beta rays from radioactive substances, have immensely more energy than is stored in the individual binding of atoms in chemical compounds, so that radiation is nearly always destructive of complex molecular structures, destructive that is of biological organization and hence also destructive on the macro-scale. X rays and gamma rays release high energy electrons from the materials in which they are absorbed and these charged particles, similar in nature to the beta rays of radioactive substances, are the effective agents of biological action. Neutrons act in a more complex way, but much of their effect, if initially energetic, is brought about by collision with hydrogen nuclei, setting them in recoil motion. Neutrons may also enter the nuclei of atoms, thus causing an instability which expresses itself, as does all radioactivity, in the subsequent breakup of the unstable atom with an accompanying emission of radiation.

Some elementary physical properties of the radiations, such as their penetrating power in tissues, are very variable as between different particles. They also define the probable primary biological effect of the radiation. Thus natural alpha rays travel only very short distances, say 20 to 50 microns (μ), a few cell diameters, in soft tissues and even less in dense bone. It follows that alpha-ray sources external to the body, since the rays hardly penetrate the skin, are of little importance. Should, however an alpha-ray emitting radioactive material be ingested or inhaled (as, for example, when radium luminizers licked their brushes or industrial workers breathe air containing plutonium 239) then the material, which may also enter the blood stream via wounds, will be metabolized according to the chemical nature and valency state of the particular element involved. It will then circulate around the body until caught up in a particular tissue which it thus proceeds to irradiate, though in the case of alpha-ray emitters this irradiation will be confined to a few cells in the immediate neighbourhood of the active material. If the radioactive substance emits beta rays these normally travel much further in soft tissues, perhaps a few millimetres or even a centimetre from their origin, thus irradiating more cells per particle but leaving less energy in each cell through which they pass.

The distribution of a given substance, whether active or inactive, in the body thus depends upon its chemical nature. Radioactive strontium, for example, behaves like stable or radioactive calcium and is selectively taken up in bone, which is thereby irradiated. Tissues in rapid growth or development tend to utilize more material whether stable or radioactive, thus providing the reason for our particular anxiety about the irradiation of the bones of growing children by strontium 90, but also providing us with the possibility of selective irradiation and destruction of malignant disease by beta-ray emitting materials.

High energy X and gamma rays penetrate tens of centimetres or even metres in soft tissues so that an external X or gamma-ray source (such as a 4 meV linear accelerator or a strong cobalt 60 source) may give essentially 'whole-body radiation'.

It follows that although the biological effects of all ionizing radiations are essentially similar, in practical situations the damage may be distributed throughout the body in very different ways, depending on the chemical nature of the emitter and properties of the rays emitted. Sometimes, as in medical practice, the geometrical pattern of irradiation is deliberately decided by choice of external conditions, perhaps by a radiotherapist who wishes to irradiate a tumour and spare normal tissue, or by a diagnostician examining an abdomen and yet at the same time trying to avoid direct irradiation of gonads. The protection problems in industry vary from the local irradiation of a lung by inhaled radioactive particles to whole-body irradiation by gamma rays or neutrons from a nuclear reactor. Of course this geometrical limitation of the primary beam of radiation does not necessarily limit the field of the biological consequences. The genetic effects of radiation depend primarily upon the dose to gonads, but the effects may be apparent in individuals of the next generation. The irradiation of the pituitary gland may bring in its train serious hormonal unbalance, and some of the most important changes due to heavy irradiation result from an interference with blood supply and may be observed at a distance from the directly irradiated site.

Very occasionally we encounter a material effectively taken up by metabolic processes in a specific organ or tissue as, for example, iodine in the thyroid. Since isotopes of iodine usually emit only beta rays or gamma rays of low effective penetration, the irradiation due to them is largely confined to that gland. Such selective metabolism is rare but useful when it occurs. Sufficient quantities of iodine may be administered to a patient to treat hyperthyroidism or malignant disease. Alternatively, very small quantities of radioactive iodine, readily detected by modern methods, may be introduced by injection or ingestion, so that by studying its rate of uptake in the thyroid or its excretion in urine or saliva, useful information may be obtained concerning the patient's physiological condition. It should be noted that even in the case of a relatively specific uptake such as this, attention must be given to possible irradiation of other tissues, as for example kidney or blood, since the radioactive material moves about on its way to resynthesis and excretion. Such consideration of general irradiation is particularly important for materials such as caesium 137. Caesium is retained at a number of sites in the body, particularly muscle and other soft tissues and so administers a widely spread internal dose of gamma rays. The same is true of sodium 24 and also of a radioactive isotope of potassium (K40) naturally present in all of us, even those who have not been exposed to artificial radioactive materials. From a physico-chemical point of view each radioactive substance presents a complex spatial and temporal pattern of material movement and consequent irradiation which it is often hard to unravel. Commencing perhaps in a circumscribed volume around a site of injection or ingestion the material may be carried in the blood stream to distant organs in which it may reside for varying lengths of time. Later it may be gradually eliminated in fæces, urine or sweat, saliva or exhaled air, thus irradiating not only specific organs but metabolic pathways of great importance. The pattern of radiation exposure is not necessarily the same as the pattern of movement and distribution of the active material in the body, though related to it, and deducable from it by fairly simple mathematical techniques.

The physical problems are, however, trivial compared to those associated with the definition and quantitation of the resulting biological effects. The relationship between radiation dose and biological effect in a given organ containing the radioactive material is usually complex, and the body as an integrated whole may suffer secondary damage as the result of the destruction or malfunction of a single vital organ. It seems frequently to happen that the overall effects are dominated by those in one particular organ such as the bone marrow (the blood-forming organ), the gut or the gonads. This organ is often known as the 'critical organ' and in a desperate effort at simplification in our attempt to guess safe levels of a given material, attention is essentially concentrated on this organ alone.

We shall see that many radiation problems arise from the power of ionizing radiations to produce changes in cell nuclei, thus producing mutation of genes and genetic effects. When one begins to try to assess the effects on a whole human population of the irradiation of individual gonads, one begins to realize that the presence of radioactive material in the environment may, indeed, give rise to complex and puzzling situations.

Yet it is only fair to add that we probably know more about the distribution in the human body of radioactive materials and their radiations than we know about any other noxious agent. The relative simplicity of nuclear phenomena as compared to chemical, and the fairly high degree of understanding that we have of nuclear phenomena and radiation make the prediction and control of the hazards more straightforward. I also suspect that more attention has been given to this particular hazard than has been devoted to other fields, certainly during the last few years. We do at least know that the radiation we detect in the body after the introduction of appreciable amounts of radioactive materials is the proximate cause of the biological damage and we can sometimes measure its amount with sufficient accuracy to enable biological consequence to be roughly predicted. On the other hand, a complex organic molecule introduced into the body may eventually produce malignant disease, but will almost certainly undergo a series of metabolic changes, so that the real 'carcinogenic agent' is a matter of good chemical speculation. Moreover, the absolute amounts of such material in the body as a whole or at specific sites at which tumours appear, are usually quite unknown. It happens that my own first experience of industrial hazard was in the field of chemical carcinogens, and I have tried to study the generalities of chemical toxicity in the hope of finding helpful analogies with the radiation problems. I have thus been constantly reminded of detailed knowledge in the radiation field, crude though it is, compared to the relative absence of detailed knowledge in others. This situation stems largely from the elaborate and extremely sensitive physical techniques which have been developed in the last few years to measure radiation and assay radioactive materials and their concentrations even in the living body. By making appropriate external or internal observations supplemented by the study of biopsy samples of tissues, body fluids, excreta and post mortem material, we may often build up a picture of the metabolism involved. 'Scanners' enable us to form visual patterns of distributions of radioactive materials in the living body and there is at the moment great interest in elaborate pinhole cameras with powerful electronic detectors which enable a limited region to be 'seen' and movements of radioactive materials followed by eye. Doubtless much development making use of advanced television and radio-communication technology will occur in this field during the next few years. Let me, however, hasten to add that our lack of knowledge of the detailed pattern of metabolism of radioactive materials in the human body is still the first bar to progress in making wise decisions as to utilization in safety. The second is basic biological ignorance.

One of the obvious characteristics of any enquiry involving the physical sciences, and ours must strongly partake of such characteristic, is its emphasis on number, on amount. Qualitative concepts will not suffice. We are interested not merely in the nature of radiation and its interactions, but in how much radiation is involved in a particular event. It is obvious from even casual observation that, as with other noxious agents, the larger the amount of radiation administered the more serious the biological effects produced.

Radiation is a form of energy and is therefore measurable in the appropriate units, but the amounts involved in producing biological effects are often too small for us to carry out the measurement at all readily. The specification of radiation for biological and medical purposes is, however, full of pitfalls. Moreover, the choice of a system of units for measuring radiations in medicine seemed to some to be the most boring of scientific disciplines and to others a fascinating set of decisions involving many human as well as scientific judgements. Needless to say, I stand among the second group.

We have good human as well as scientific cause to follow the injunctions of Deuteronomy (xxv, 14–15): 'Thou shalt not have in thine house divers measures, a great and a small. But thou shalt have a perfect and just weight, a perfect and just measure shalt thou have; that thy days may be lengthened in the land which the Lord thy God giveth thee'. The choice of a 'perfect and just measure' for radiation is not easy and perhaps the last phrase looks ominously like a reference to radiation life-shortening!

I personally cannot forget easily the patients whom I saw irradiated therapeutically with low-voltage X rays some

40 years ago, at a time when no system of measurement had been agreed and no clinician could in any real sense transfer even part of his experience to another or even compare his own from day to day. Mistakes and tragedies are very easily obscured in talk of 'hyper-sensitivity' and 'idiosyncrasy'. We were in the position of those administering dangerous drugs and having no balance to weigh them with, or worse still, balances changing erratically in an unknown way from moment to moment. No one was better aware of this situation than Rock Carling, or tried harder via the Radium Commission to insist on the necessity of acceptable physical standardization.[4] Some workers turned to radium, the most used radioactive substance of those days, as a standard, for at least it gave a steady output of radiation, and a scheme of dosimetry based upon time of exposure and the amount of radium afforded some basis for judgement. It turned out, however, that the geometrical factors of irradiation were more troublesome and complex than initially realized.

During the years 1920 to 1930 a system of measurement based on the electrical conductivity produced in air under the action of X rays was established and later extended to gamma rays. It was somewhat arbitrarily chosen, but for reasons we need not discuss here corresponded fairly well to a measurement of the energy absorbed in soft tissues and formed the basis of the unit named after the discoverer of X rays, the röntgen.

Various difficulties arose as the voltage applied to X ray tubes increased from perhaps 100 keV to 20 meV in our endeavour to produce more and more penetrating X rays, thus enabling us to treat more deeply-seated tumours with less effects on the skin, but these difficulties were met rather by refinement of concept and definition than by fundamentally new approaches. All of this experience provided the basis of the present-day unit of dose of radiation, the 'rad', which represents simply an energy absorption of 100 ergs per gram of tissue or other material. We should perhaps also introduce here a relative newcomer, the 'rem', which represents an attempt to weight each type of radiation according to its biological effectiveness. To fix orders of magnitude as to significance in practice, let me say that 1 rad is a fairly small dose for most medical purposes. About 300 to 500 rad absorbed throughout the whole body will produce an even chance of death in humans. Tumours and small volumes are frequently given 6,000 to 10,000 rad in the course of treatment for malignant disease. We permit 5 rad per year to occupationally exposed persons as the maximum dose they should be allowed to receive each year for a few years. We shall see in a moment that we in this country are all irradiated to the extent of about 0·1 rad per year by natural ionizing radiations. For genetic doses to the whole population we begin to think in terms of milli-rad, that is thousandths of a rad, and of upper levels of 0·3 rad or 300 milli-rad per year.

When in 1945 tremendous changes occurred in the availability and use of artificially produced radioactive materials in medicine, this system of units proved in principle surprisingly adequate. I have no doubt that our insistence 20 years previously on absorbed energy as the fundamental physical parameter to be correlated with biological effect saved years of clinical experiment and many dangerous clinical errors. The system of dosimetry was able to take in its stride the wide range of radioactive materials emitting a vast spectrum of radiations of individually characteristic, but overall varied types.

The present-day difficulties arise rather from biological and medical complexities, though micro-dosimetry still requires much further development. We all know that the biological effect of radiation, in general, increases with the dose given, but perhaps in our naive innocence those of us responsible for the choice of units before the growth of radiobiology to its present somewhat inchoate mass, hoped for simple quantitative correlations between clear-cut 'biological effect' and energy absorbed per unit mass of tissue. We were to be disillusioned, for first of all it turned out that though qualitatively similar, the magnitude of the effect per unit dose depended on a variety of factors such as volume of tissue irradiated, type of cell irradiated and the point in its cycle of division, on the time-spacing of irradiation, on the presence or relative absence of oxygen as well as on the precise pattern of micro-concentrations of energy, and a host of other factors. Again, the biological effect of radiation came to mean to the theorist not an 'effect' but the 'probability of an effect', as we realized that the quantum nature of radiation implied that a small object in a low dose field stood a good chance of not being irradiated at all in any real sense of the term. The ionizing events might well be concentrated around but not in the cellular target. We became involved in discussions of the form of the dose-response relationship. Was the 'effect' proportional to dose or did it show a 'threshold' below which nothing was observable? Alternatively, as seemed probable, were there other more complex relations to be found between a dose and its effect? We began to create naive theories (and all our theories may still be classified this way) based upon the idea of a sensitive 'region' within a cell whose destruction or alteration brought about the biological effect. This was a very important concept though at the moment such simple theories are a little unfashionable. They have had to be modified to take into account the more remote secondary chemical effects of a 'hit' which may have diffused throughout the cell. Energy is handed in a complex way around a cell. The chain breaks at the weakest link, not necessarily where it is pulled. The new knowledge on cellular micro-organization obtained by the use of the electron microscope has hardly as yet been integrated into any general picture of radiation damage. The mobility of so-called genetic messenger materials and their metabolites still further widen and complicate the theoretical picture. We have begun to talk learnedly (I fear with Whitehead's dreaded 'misty profundity') of 'information', 'organization' and 'entropy' in biological systems. There is no comprehensive overall theory of radiation damage at the subcellular level at the present time. How could there be, until there is a satisfactory overall picture of normal cellular structure and metabolism, and this certainly is as yet far removed? Besides, radiation often only pulls triggers. The direct absorption of one rad in soft tissues would only bring about a direct rise of temperature of about two millionths of a degree centigrade. Yet a dose of a few hundred rad causing a direct rise of only a few ten thousandths of a degree centigrade, may set in train biological responses causing rises of temperature of thousands of times this amount. The energy released in whole intact animals by biological reaction to ionizing radiation is overwhelmingly from chemical reactions set in train and only a very small fraction of a percent from the radiation directly.

This is not, however, true on the cellular or subcellular scale and, since such apparent contradictions pervade the whole interpretation of radiation damage, it may be wise to treat this point in a little more detail.

Let us think of an alpha particle having an energy of 5 meV (8·0 $\times$ 10^{-6} ergs). This particle will only penetrate about 30 micron (μ) in soft tissues. Its track may be thought of as having a cross-section of perhaps 0·01 μ^2. The energy absorbed in this minute volume (0·3 μ^3) is very high and equivalent to the enormous dose of a quarter of a million rad in this very small volume. This clearly would raise the temperature in the immediate vicinity of the track very considerably and we see the origin of the old 'point-heat' theory of biological damage, popular 40 years ago. One must realize, however, that the 'volume' concerned is only that of a small fraction of a single cell. The damage is intense but local. Even if we admit that the five cells or so through which the alpha particle passes might be killed, would this necessarily be of any consequence to the whole organism? The body sheds from gastric mucosæ and lung an enormous number of cells, perhaps 10^{12} per day. Can five extra matter? We frequently meet this dilemma. Imagine a radioactive particle breathed in and lodged in the lung, subsequently emitting alpha or soft beta rays. There may be great concentration of radiation absorption in its immediate vicinity. The particle may move on a sheet of mucous material set in motion by ciliary action and so spread its effect. Everything depends on what we mean by dose and upon the precise micro-biological life history of the particle. We are faced with the question whether the dose in a microscopic volume of a single cell or group of cells is the important parameter in assessing biological damage or should we consider the mean, usually very small dose, in the whole tissue or organ? There can be no single simple answer. We may easily imagine that if by chance a vital cell at an important moment in its life history, as for instance a sperm about to enter an ovum and to fertilize it, is affected by an alpha or beta particle being thereby either killed or perhaps worse, so changed as to suffer a mutation of one of its genes, then this minute event could be of consequence throughout a whole human life and indeed transmitted into the racial germ plasm as a deleterious permanency. The corresponding event during an X-ray examination of a pregnant woman could cause an alteration leading to leukæmia in her offspring. We are dealing not with inevitable 'effects' but remote possibilities. The probability of such an event is minute, but the presiding goddess is Tyche, the ungodly goddess with a double face, and not Artemis. We must give her as little encouragement as possible.

So far, we have considered only the measurement of the radiations, but some thought must also be given to the specification of amount of radioactive material. It might reasonably have been assumed that the amount of a radioactive substance would be expressed simply by its weight, but this procedure would be very inconvenient. All radioactive substances are disintegrating spontaneously and randomly and hence decreasing in amount with time, but the disintegration rate (the chance that an atom will disintegrate within the next unit of time) is extremely variable as between different substances. Some atomic species have an even chance of disintegrating in micro-micro-seconds, while others may persist on the average for thousands of millions of years. Different isotopes of the same element often have extremely different rates of disintegration.

From the point of view of biological or even physical effects the important quantity concerning a radioactive material is the radiation emitted in a given time, in its turn associated with the number of atoms disintegrating in that time. If the chance of disintegration in a given time of a particular kind of atom is low then to obtain a given overall disintegration rate the total number of atoms required must be correspondingly increased. It was, therefore, decided after much argument to use as a standard of amount of radioactivity the amount of any substance having the same rate of disintegration as one gram of radium, that is $3 \cdot 700 \times 10^{10}$ disintegrations per second. This amount of any material is now called a 'curie'. For most purposes it represents a large amount. In medical or protection problems we frequently have to deal with a milli-curie (mc), which is one thousandth of a curie, or a micro-curie (μc), which is one millionth of a curie. In studies of natural and other environmental materials one millionth again of this quantity represents a useful order of magnitude, that is 1 micro-microcurie (1 $\mu\mu$c) or 1 pica-curie (1 pc). This extremely small amount of radioactive material suffers only $2 \cdot 2$ atomic disintegrations per minute and it is easy to show that the number of atoms in a pica-curie of many radio-active substances is quite small. Our soft tissues contain only about a single atom of polonium 210 on the average in half a million living cells. One must, however, be a little wary of this argument for there is evidence that some types of atoms, for example polonium, tend to be located in particular rare kinds of cells in a tissue, thus providing a possible mechanism of significant action by only a few atoms.

We have little difficulty with recent techniques in detecting and identifying these extremely small concentrations, which nevertheless deliver measurable amounts of radiation to human tissues, even when we estimate the effect throughout the whole mass. One sometimes wonders whether the astonishing sensitivity of modern physical techniques in detecting single atomic events is not a trap. We can detect so very little radioactivity, but to assess its significance or absence of significance is quite another matter. I personally have found the attempt to gauge the significance of atomic and sub-atomic events in a macroscopic problem, fascinating but full of imaginative pitfalls.

To sum up this brief and certainly inadequate summary of the physical aspects of ionizing radiations, we are left with a picture of microscopic complex structures subject to local disruption as ionizing events occur at random throughout their volumes. Radiation is *par excellence* an indiscriminate agent. At large doses even very small microstructures in cells stand a high chance of immediate disruption, but as the radiation dose is reduced, larger and larger regions are left unaffected by these primary events. The radiation due to radioactive materials in tissues is subject to a double randomness. At very low concentrations there may be a random element in the distribution of the atoms among the cells of the tissue or organism, coupled with a second chance phenomenon in the distribution of the ionization resulting from its radiations. If the material is present in large amounts every cell may harbour numbers of the intruders, but as we reduce the amount the majority of cells may contain no radioactive atoms of the given species. The only exception among the naturally occurring material seems to be potassium 40, five million atoms on the average present per cell, and disintegrating at the rate of about five per minute for every gram of soft tissue, thus contributing one of the major fractions of human natural irradiation.

As to the resulting biological effects of radiation, we must visualize the bombardment of a highly organized active community which reacts to repair the damage and already has a high 'turnover' of workers. The loss of a few more individuals may be unimportant, but the loss of a large number quite devastating. Moreover, the maiming or death of key personnel may have far-reaching effects throughout the community. The physical micro-structures embodying vital functions will have very varying degrees of stability and sensitivity. No microbiological structure will, however, withstand a direct hit, but some will be destroyed at a greater distance from such a hit than others. When repair begins the reconstruction of the life of the community may be badly disrupted or perturbed not only by mechanical debris, but by the distortion of vital messages as to how the repair is to be effected and the prevention of the arrival of essential material. Survival of the individual microscopic unit is a matter of chance, but the overall severity of the attack determines that chance. The biological effect depends on the dose. Those conversant with Civil Defence, another of Rock Carling's enthusiasms, will have little difficulty in visualizing the microscopic cellular community under attack.

Chapter 2

THE BIOLOGICAL EFFECTS OF
RADIATION, SOMATIC AND GENETIC

We have seen that the micro-physical phenomena underlying the effects of ionizing radiation are in a sense indiscriminate and capricious and it is, therefore, not surprising that the biological outcome of heavy irradiation is complex and of great variety. Every system of the body, every control mechanism, every tissue, every structure, is at risk and it is by no means easy even to make the decision how to decide what tissues are to be regarded as most sensitive.

It would be ridiculous to attempt here a summary of present-day knowledge of the effects of radiation, particularly as the reader may find excellent accounts in recent reports by the Medical Research Council,[5, 6] the United Nations Scientific Committee on the Effects of Atomic Radiation,[7] and many other individual publications. The effects of practical significance are set out in publications by the International Commission on Radiological Protection,[8] and I shall, therefore, merely attempt some individual comment on one or two important issues.

First, as to the origin of information upon which we must make our judgements. The science of radiobiology has contributed greatly and may in time do so even more significantly in the study of the effects of radiations on human beings. It must be admitted that its light is at present often dim and wavering and that sometimes we are distracted by the flashing of too many lights simultaneously. Much of our

35

information is, therefore, still derived from medical experience. Both X rays and gamma rays have been used for many years in the treatment of disease, mainly cancer, and this experience has been valuable in yielding information on the general effects of radiation on many different tissues. Radiotherapy has been stigmatized as empirical or worse. I can sometimes see why, but at least if one wishes to know the effects of radiation on human beings one should look at irradiated human beings. The circumstances of radiotherapy normally imply the careful collimation of beams of radiation to prescribed and selected tissues and this type of experience has the advantage that these irradiations are carefully controlled and the doses of radiation reasonably accurately known. It has the limitation of being concerned with the effects observed on pathological conditions and care must be exercised in extrapolating to 'normal' individuals, though unfortunately much 'normal' tissue may be irradiated. More caution is perhaps required in extrapolating to 'whole-body irradiation'. Definite destructive effects are aimed at in radiotherapy and the doses are, therefore, relatively very high whereas our most troublesome protection problems usually relate to very low doses and large populations. We are, therefore, left with the problem of deducing the effects of very small doses per head of a very large population from the observed dramatic effects of a large dose on one or two individuals.

The therapeutic and diagnostic uses of radioactive isotopes have provided much data and stimulated much research into the effects of radioactivity within the body. It may be that the increasing use of very small quantities of radioactive materials as tracers or in diagnostic investigations will provide equally useful information on the absence of significant effect of these materials in small quantities. This is, of course, a very important practical matter since the use of volunteers in such investigations has rightly hitherto been regarded with suspicion and treated with caution, though an obvious way of obtaining information of the greatest possible utility. Increasingly such investigations can be carried out with amounts of radioactive material little above those naturally present in the human body and thus provide one of the main incentives to the development of what may seem absurdly sensitive equipment.

A second source of information regarding radiation effects is the study of persons involved in known occupational hazards, as for example medical radiological workers, painters of luminous dials, miners working radioactive ores, or the now classical Schneeberg miners. This experience is unfortunately being supplemented by more modern information from accidents occurring in or around nuclear reactors or critical assemblies. For instance, six accidents (one at a military installation at Lockport, New York, one at the Y12 plant at Oak Ridge, three at Los Alamos, U.S.A., and one at Vinca, Yugoslavia) occurring during recent years, mostly through ignorance of hazards or fortuitous conjunction of several unrelated factors, have been carefully studied.[9] They underlined the difficulties of assessing dosimetry in the complex circumstances of an accident, and have certainly stimulated research into such fields as the treatment of acute radiation injury, the irradiation of patients in preparation for kidney transplantation, and the treatment of leukæmia by combined irradiation and bone marrow transfusion. A major contribution of irradiation to the study of immunity and organ transplantation might well be counted some day as one of its most valuable contributions to human welfare.

We naturally turn next to experience of the effects of nuclear explosions.[10] Atomic bomb explosions bring widespread destruction and casualties, mostly caused by blast and fire, but about one-fifth of the total casualties are usually thought to be due to gamma and neutron exposure. The dosimetry, though studied in great detail, must necessarily be confused and inaccurate. The immediate and long-term effects on survivors have been carefully studied and have contributed significantly to our knowledge of radiation effects, particularly perhaps in relation to genetic effects and the time-incidence and risk of leukæmia as well as the production of other malignant disease in the irradiated population. In view of the long latent period involved such investigations are necessarily long-term projects, and jubilation that so far little has been seen could prove premature. These, then, are the main sources of our knowledge.

The biological effects themselves may be roughly classified into those affecting irradiated individuals only and those affecting their genetic material and, therefore, liable to transmission to offspring. The line is difficult to draw precisely, since fertility and length of life, circumstances affecting the probability of transmission of gene changes to future generations, are affected by heavy irradiation. Evolutionary theory shows how small changes of fertility may have considerable consequence in defining subsequent gene frequency in a given population.

The irradiated 'unit' must now be regarded as the whole

population, but I personally am one of those who see close analogies between 'somatic' and 'genetic' effects. It may even be that so-called 'somatic mutation' is an important factor in determining biological injury, as for example carcinogenesis, in an irradiated individual. In the same line of thought, some years ago I proposed a system of dosimetry based on a quantity I called 'integral dose' which tried to take into account the mass of tissue, that is roughly the number of cells at risk, as well as dose in its exact sense. I still suspect that this approach is a useful one, particularly in the study of induced malignancy, though it arose as a result of investigation of change of field-size in radiotherapy.

The precise biological effects of an irradiation depend upon many circumstances. The main factors determining somatic effects are probably magnitude of dose, extent of the body irradiated, the part of the body irradiated, the type of radiation and its distribution in the body, the age of the individual and the time-pattern of irradiation, that is whether the radiation is given in a single short time or divided into fractions and administered over varying periods. The analogy between the administration of radiation and of drugs has, of course, often been noted and theoretical discussions of quantum effects for radiation may often be paralleled by the significance of fixation of key drug-molecules at selected sites in cells.

The effects of large doses to the whole body are well known. The initial nausea, vomiting and diarrhœa, the apparent recovery for a few days and subsequent recurrence of the symptoms perhaps ten days later if the dose has been sufficiently large, have often been described. Such effects are to be expected, however, only after heavy exposure due to gross accident in the vicinity of X-ray equipment, radioactive sources or nuclear reactors, or of course immediately following atomic bombing. In peace-time they are liable to affect very few individuals in very special circumstances and might, therefore, be regarded as in the same category as other major personal catastrophes.

From these accidents involving doses of some hundreds of rad in a short time to much of the body we turn to the commoner problem of high doses, again perhaps hundreds of rad, given accidentally to limited portions of the body, as to the hands of workers with X-ray crystallographic units. The effects may be severe and result in localized necrosis with all that this implies. Again, relatively few people are at risk.

One of the main problems in industrial radiography is the accidental administration of smaller doses repeated at relatively short time intervals. We have now to consider the possibility of long-term blood changes including the induction of leukæmia.

Nowadays great emphasis is laid on the possible effects of small doses of radiation to which the whole or an appreciable fraction of the population is potentially exposed. The knowledge that a particular effect *can* be produced by a sufficient quantity of radiation is an insufficient basis in itself for asserting that this effect *will* develop as a result of a particular exposure. The knowledge that carbon monoxide is a deadly poison is not in itself a sufficient basis for estimation of the effects of badly ventilated kitchens or even for the suggestion to abolish gas central heating. For the precise study of radiation risk, as for example the induction of a particular disease, it is necessary to estimate from natural mortality statistics the incidence of the disease in the absence of exposure to radiation (additional to that from natural sources), and then to compare this figure with the incidence of the same condition in a population which has been exposed to extra radiation. It will be noted that we have no idea who will be the victims, but merely how many there might be. We note the significance of the study of the usual level of natural radiation as a basis for the estimation of what may be expected from increased natural or artificial exposure. We see, too, that if the national incidence of a given disease is low and possibly changing owing to quite different social circumstance, it may be extremely difficult to establish that a small additional incidence of that disease is due to a particular cause such as man-made radiation. It is only against a very stable background that a small increase can be unequivocally demonstrated. These considerations apply, for example, to one of the most debated problems, namely that of leukæmia, to which we now turn. As a physicist I find myself in some embarrassment here and can only refer the reader to the literature, as for example to Dr. Loutit's excellent and lively discussion in his book *Irradiation of Mice and Men*.[11]

In many countries the recorded death rates from leukæmia have shown a steady rise in recent years, some rise possibly due to improved diagnosis, though there seems evidence of a real increase. Arguing from animal studies, bomb victims, and radiotherapeutic experience, there can be no reasonable doubt that radiation can 'cause' leukæmia in the sense that a dose of radiation increases the probability of its occurrence, but the precise mechanism and the correlation of this knowledge with recent advances as to the significance of viruses in leukæmia is still unsure. Some of the problems may be illustrated by valuable investigations in this field involving the study of patients suffering from ankylosing spondylitis.[12] Patients, often active young men suffering from this very painful and crippling disease, benefit by X-ray treatment during which the whole spine, or part of it, is irradiated. In most cases pain and stiffness are relieved and general health improved. Many of the patients return to productive work. An analysis of the results of treatment of some 14,000 patients showed that 38 developed leukæmia, an incidence about ten times greater than would have been expected from the national death rate over the same period. There are, of course, possible explanations in terms of greater frequency of occurrence of leukæmia among those suffering from ankylosing spondylitis than in the normal population, though control studies show no such effect. Alternatively, spondylitis might in some way increase the patients' susceptibility to leukæmia on irradiation. It seems that the dose to the spinal marrow needed to double the expected incidence of leukæmia (i.e. increase it by 0·5 cases per 10,000 men annually) is roughly 94 rad. If all the red marrow had been irradiated this dose might have been smaller, say 30 to 50 rad. The observations mean that 0·3 per cent of the men treated with relatively enormous doses of radiation develop leukæmia. With lower doses, probably sufficient in many cases, the risk would, of course, have been proportionally reduced. Was it not worth that risk?

We see how different these numbers appear as we look from varying points of view. Ten times the normal risk of leukæmia looks pretty severe. If we note that only 0·3 per cent of the men treated suffered from the disease we feel a little less depressed. If we take the view of the therapist that the 'improvement to be expected from this form of therapy of a crippling and painful disease is so much greater than from any other that it should be given at the earliest opportunity', we have obviously moved to the other end of the scale of opinions. The Report of the Adrian Committee on Radiological Hazards to Patients[13] concluded that 'the benefits of radiotherapy for this serious and disabling disease are great and far outweigh any radiological hazard both genetic and somatic', but nevertheless very rightly suggested as low doses as possible and the use of male gonad shields.

Perhaps this example illustrates the problem of balancing good and evil effects of radiation. Here fortunately we have a clearly established gain from radiation and one can balance effects. It is not always so. We do not meet here the delicate balancing of 'loss' to unfortunate individuals selected at random against a problematic gain to a different whole population.

We shall see later that the amount of radiation received in the bone marrow from natural radiation background by an Englishman of the average age of the men studied is about 5 rad. If the induction of leukæmia by radiation is the result of the production of a mutation in a somatic cell, then it may be that natural background radiation is responsible for a proportion of genetic mutation and of leukæmia. If we assume no 'threshold' and a linear relationship with dose the spondylitic data suggest that some 5 per cent of naturally occurring leukæmia is, in fact, due to background radiation, but dose-rate effects and the different nature of the radiations make these estimates uncertain.

Perhaps the most formidable of all tasks confronting anyone writing about radiation and health is to attempt a brief summary of the genetic effects of radiation. So much has been written authoritatively, recklessly, tendentiously, politically, cautiously, even scientifically, and yet the fundamental uncertainty remains.

Let us merely recall[14] that the hereditary material is contained in the cell in chromosomes present in pairs, one member of maternal and the other of paternal origin. These chromosomes are composed of units known as genes, liable to 'spontaneous' or 'forced' mutation. Some genes produce a given bodily trait when paired with like or unlike partners; they are 'dominant'. Other genes produce their effect only when paired with similar partners; they are 'recessive'. But I should warn that the distinction is much less clear-cut than here suggested. Genes, originally often thought of as individual self-contained units, have important interactions on each other and a single gene is not necessarily responsible for a given trait which may be produced by other combinations of genes. Radiation damages these gene structures only when the sex organs are themselves irradiated so that the dose to those organs becomes the primary consideration when we attempt to think of the genetic consequence of radiation to a population.

Some of the most important scientific advance of our generation concerns the chemical structure of genes and for the first time we have some inkling of how they function as carriers of heredity. The most important constituent of genes is an extraordinary substance known as desoxyribo-nucleic acid (DNA). Its molecules are long fibres, often compared to the tapes upon which information is printed to control computers. These molecules do almost certainly carry in code the instructions to the cell for all its vital functions of living, growing and dividing. Their incredible efficiency is illustrated by pointing out that all the chromosomes present initially in the fertilized eggs from which the present world population developed would occupy only the volume of an aspirin tablet.

These gene structures are self-duplicating from relatively simple molecules, thus forming the new 46 chromosomes of the normal human living cell. There are probably hundreds of thousands of genes per chromosome. All the genes act together to bring about development, a given gene perhaps synthesizing one or more enzymes to facilitate particular chemical reactions. If the gene is destroyed or altered the cell may perform some function imperfectly or die. The perpetuation of gene mutation is easily imagined as resulting from a mistake in the coded sequence of nucleotides within the gene. Clearly the destruction wrought by an ionizing event in the neighbourhood of a gene may break or distort the DNA and so cause an error. The mutated gene during the course of subsequent gene and chromosome duplication reproduces itself in the altered form and so the change is transmitted to the next generation.

Ordinarily the genes reproduce themselves with astonishing precision and only very rarely mutate, the chances of their doing so spontaneously being probably to be measured in a few hundred thousands to one chance against. This is a fairly small chance. If we put twenty balls into a bag, ten of which are white and ten red, and select at random ten balls, the chance of selecting all white or all red is about the same (5×10^{-6}) as this chance of mutation.

Thus in one form of dwarfism about 4 per hundred thousand sex cells produced by normal persons carry the necessary deleterious gene. Unfortunately mutations which result in degenerative changes, hereditary disease or lethality are far more frequent than mutations which are potentially or actually useful. Gene mutation may be brought about by a wide variety of causes, including many chemical substances (mutagens), heat and other physical agents such as radiation.

When we turn to the quantitative aspects of genetics and radiation important results emerge. All kinds of ionizing radiations cause mutations, though there is some difference in the mutation rate per ionization with the type of radiation. It seems that within a wide range of circumstances and doses the number of point mutations induced is the same regardless of whether the exposure takes a long or short time, provided the same total dose is given.

The critical question is whether the effect is strictly proportional to dose. Is there a 'threshold' below which no effect is observed? Can recovery from radiation injury of this kind take place?

With physiological damage such as radiation burns, sickness or erythema, there exists a minimal amount (a threshold) and a critical intensity. If the amount or rate is below this minimum there is no obvious effect. Healing processes can within limits counterbalance the effects of radiation in this type of system, but for genetic damage there seems to be little in the way of healing processes. Medical men, largely no doubt because of emphasis on physiology in their training, find it difficult to visualize a biological event in which ability to heal or revert to normal is lacking. It may well be that they are to some extent right, for there is now evidence that at low dose-rates part of the damage caused by radiation to genetic material can undergo a process of repair. At high dose-rates the mechanism leading to repair may well be inhibited. We must await much more research in this obviously vital subject which affects profoundly our views of probable significance of ionizing radiation. We must remember that many chemical substances can also cause mutations, perhaps more subtle and selective than by radiation but the basic chemistry is only just beginning to be understood. Various other changes of physical environment can lead to change of mutation rate, as for example temperature, since rise of temperature generally raises spontaneous mutation rate. This is evidently a reflection of a fundamental instability and the probability of change of molecular configuration as a result of molecular movements in genes and chromosomes.

So much for the individual gamete, that is reproductive cell, but the main problems of radiation genetics are concerned with whole populations.

Each generation of human beings is in a sense the cross-section at a particular moment of an immortal germ plasm having a given spectrum of genes and subject to the physical and chemical influences of its environment. As this environment changes so does the supply of a particular gene alter from generation to generation and build up to a level determined by many factors, but principally by its rate of supply, its rate of transmission from generation to generation and its rate of elimination via defective individuals. The precise details of this build-up are dependent upon the type of gene, as for instance whether it is dominant or recessive. In some instances recessive genes may have beneficial effects in particular environments so far as fertility or resistance to a particular disease is concerned, and may in unsuspected ways tend to balance the effect of depletion. In this way we may explain the presence in some populations of a much larger number of a particular type of gene than we would have expected from its probable rate of production.

In an equilibrium population a fundamental theorem of mathematical genetics shows how neither dominant nor recessive genes will increase or decrease in frequency. A dominant gene does not tend to displace the recessive. The overall frequency of genes tends to be transmitted from generation to generation. This is, however, obviously only correct if genes do not change by mutation and that carriers of different genes leave on the average the same number of offspring. Also, that no immigration or emigration brings in or removes one gene in preference to another and, finally, that the population is large enough so that the accidental variation of gene frequency may be ignored.

We thus reach the idea of genetic equilibrium which may be disturbed by an increase of deleterious genes in a particular generation, a change in the rate of transference of the genes, or their rate of removal. The latter might, for example, be changed by improved social services. Another important factor is mean age at marriage, since some mutation rates are undoubtedly correlated with parental age. Perhaps the earlier age of marriage of recent years is in some instances as important a factor as radiation. A harmful gene that comes into a population eventually has to be removed. The actual number of people carrying a recessive gene is often far greater than those showing an effect. For instance, imagine 50 persons in the United Kingdom or one person per million dying in each generation (30 years) from a particular type of recessive lethal mutation. This represents an average of 2 deaths per year and may seem a very rare disease, but it is easily shown that that means that roughly 1 person in 500 carries the harmful gene so that in the population of the United Kingdom the number of persons enjoying apparently normal health but carrying the lethal gene is about 100,000. Thus the population contains large numbers of genes for recessive hereditary diseases, malfunctions and weaknesses of all kinds. This is its 'genetic load'. We note again the difficulty of defining 'health'. What percentage of perfect health is to be ascribed to the carrier of a particular recessive deleterious gene showing no clinical symptoms? As a result of past experience of the race each of us carries a load of recessive mutations awaiting their chance to express themselves, but the size and composition of this genetic load in human populations cannot at present be estimated precisely. We may be sure that excess irradiation will increase it, hence the low limits of radiation suggested for whole populations.

There has been much discussion of the so-called 'doubling dose', namely, the dose required to double the spontaneous mutation rate. It lies probably around 30 rad, but is variable from gene to gene even in the same chromosome and it is not certain that the concept is now very useful. Recent research has emphasized the production of chromosome aberrations by radiation as opposed to gene mutation and opened up interesting correlations between disease and chromosome abnormality.

It is frequently assumed that a given amount of radiation has the same genetic effect on a population whether a fairly large dose is given to a few individuals or a correspondingly smaller amount to a larger number of individuals, but this is clearly a first simple assumption and the subsequent history of an initial small 'pool' of radiation-affected genes may be different from the effects of more general irradiation. It will be noted that inasmuch as the obvious effect of recessive genes depends upon the chances of their being combined with similar genes, then the mating pattern of the population, as for example the fraction of cousin marriages or generally the frequency of marriages between close relatives, may greatly affect the external expression of the internal deleterious situation.

In man, population structure has probably reached its maximum complexity. He inhabits the whole globe and his unity of species is manifest in any large city. Even before modern methods of transportation were commonly used, wars and human adventures had ensured that strange genes were sometimes left in faraway places. Clearly, man does not mate in a random way and this complicates our theoretical calculations. Love is blind and can often stumble only to the limits of the village or the social club. Mendelian populations are rarely sharply defined and difference in language, religion, economic status, education and profession help to subdivide a large population into smaller and smaller groups within which random mating plays a part and becomes more probable. We must put out of our mind any thought that a raising of the dose-rate will immediately cause a simple easily calculable change in the numbers of mutations or the incidence of disease or disability due to them. Some effects will be visible in the next generation. Others may take many generations, many hundreds of years, to build to equilibrium. One suspects that many other social changes may have intervened and perhaps caused much greater changes than radiation. To add to the complexity, human characteristics are often determined not by a single but by many genes acting in consort. Such traits as intelligence, height, weight at birth, are probably controlled or perhaps we should say potentiated in this way. Here radiation seems to be of less obvious significance and it has been thought that the action of radiation may be of little importance in relation to so-called continuous variation on any except an extremely long-term view. The genetic hazards of radiation seem to arise primarily from the increased frequency of simple gene mutations producing drastic effects, and these rather than the effects of continuous variation must provide the basis for our discussions as to exposure which we may regard as acceptable for human populations. There is probably nothing very urgent about the effect of ionizing radiation in relation to traits determined by multifactorial inheritance. The genetic problem is a game of chance for high stakes. It behoves us to choose our parents well from many points of view, and it seems that before consenting to be born into a family we should examine its radiation record!

Chapter 3

NATURAL RADIOACTIVITY AND ITS SIGNIFICANCE

When considering the significance of any agent possibly deleterious to health, the first question to ask is, What groups of persons have been, are, and will be, at risk? For ionizing radiation the answer is simple, 'everyone—everywhere'. We may add for good measure 'all our evolutionary ancestors', whoever they may have been. Throughout biological evolution all living organisms have been exposed to small but varying amounts of ionizing radiations. The materials by which we are surrounded and of which our bodies are made, incorporate traces of natural radioactivity. To these we have now added similar so-called 'artificial' radioactive materials of our own invention. We must make it clear that in their physical nature and biological action natural and artificial radioactive substances differ but little and are, indeed, in a number of instances identical. Man's recent nuclear activities have, for example, added extra carbon 14 to an existing stock. It is true that many natural radioactive materials are alpha emitters and that these are relatively rare among artificial radioactive isotopes which mostly emit beta and gamma rays, but there are also many beta or gamma emitters among the three main 'families' of the natural radioactive series.[15] We must, therefore, consider the two sets of radiations together, remembering that the surface of the earth has been exposed to natural radiations for some three thousand million years and to the relatively feeble artificial ones for only about 20 years.

Following the discovery of the radioactivity of a few heavy elements such as uranium, thorium or radium, it was natural that search should be made to find out if all material objects exhibited the phenomenon. It was soon established that all materials examined did, indeed, show slight traces of radioactivity. The development of modern instrumentation has amply confirmed and extended this view, the activity in many instances being due to the presence of traces of heavy naturally radioactive metals mixed with a main mass of less active material. Sometimes the activity may be due to continuing natural geophysical processes such as the incorporation throughout the biosphere of carbon 14 produced by interaction of cosmic rays with the nitrogen of the upper atmosphere.

Radioactivity is in essence a spontaneous disintegration of atomic nuclei resulting in the release of radiation and formation of new atoms which in their turn may disintegrate to give rise to further 'daughter' products, the process continuing until a member of the chain is stable and so persists indefinitely. Radioactivity expresses a fundamental complexity and instability of material things. It is not surprising, therefore, that it seems to have played a fundamental rôle in the formation of the elements and thence in the history of the world and all that is in it.

The earth, for our purposes, may be thought of as being some three thousand million years old, so that only original materials of a high order of stability can still be present. Uranium 238 and thorium 232 seem to be the 'parents' of most of the natural radioactivity. They and their daughters (including radium) form the bulk of the radioactive materials to be found in igneous, metamorphic and sedi-

mentary rocks. The sole exception of importance is a
potassium isotope of very wide occurrence, namely,
potassium 40, possibly the most important radioactive
material in the biosphere and also a main constituent of the
lithosphere. It was shown as early as 1907 by N. R. Camp-
bell that all compounds of potassium (whether derived
from potassium deposits in the earth or, for example, from
wood ash) emitted beta rays. The activity of wood had,
indeed, already been reported by Rutherford in 1903, this
being as far as I know the earliest recorded radioactivity of
'biological' material. At first the wrong isotope of potassium
was guessed to be the origin of the activity, but it is now
certain that the effective isotope is potassium 40 which also
emits gamma rays. This material contributes some 20 per
cent of the dose normally received by our soft tissues and
it is fun to demonstrate to innocent medical men the
radioactivity of normal potassium compounds and so prove
that for years they have been prescribing radioactive drugs!
About 7 atoms of potassium 40 disintegrate per second per
gram of potassium iodide. Since the human body contains
about 140 grams of potassium, its activity corresponds to
several thousand atomic disintegrations per second in our
bodies from this natural element alone. Radiopotassium
also constitutes overwhelmingly the major activity of sea
water, the total amount in the oceans being estimated at
sixty-three thousand million tons (6.3×10^{10} tons or
4.6×10^{11} curies) an amount of the same order of activities
from a nuclear power station. Since the oceans were the
scene of so much evolutionary history and the cradle of life
from Cambrian to Silurian geological periods (perhaps
200 million years) and since so many protozoa are very

small and, therefore, subject to radiation from their surroundings, potassium 40 must have been responsible for
much of the total irradiation of early living organisms.

Many hundreds of observations have been made of the
radioactive contents of igneous and sedimentary rocks with
the result that we are fairly sure of the mean content of
such rocks in the accessible regions of the earth's crust and
have good theoretical reasons for thinking that the radioactivity of the earth is very largely confined to a layer
perhaps 25 to 40 Km thick near its surface. Uranium 238
and potassium 40 are present to the extent of about 3 parts
per million, while thorium 232 tends to be about four
times as abundant on a mass basis. Oddly enough, the most
abundant known radioactive element is rubidium which
decays perhaps a little ironically to an isotope of strontium,
but its extremely low rate of disintegration and low energy
of decay make it of little practical significance. It should be
noted, too, that several billions of years ago uranium 235
(the fissile material of some atomic bombs) and potassium 40
were relatively more abundant in consequence of their
shorter half-lives. Potassium 40 was probably five times
more abundant at the time of formation of the earth's crust
than it is now. It is also probable that in the distant past
there have existed short-lived radioactive nuclei that have
long since decayed to such an extent that they are no longer
detectable in nature.

In addition to the radioactive nuclei that are probably
older than the solid earth, daughter radioactive nuclei are
continually being created in very small quantities in the
lithosphere by natural fission and the capture of natural
neutrons. Even the fission process of which our generation

is so proud was occurring naturally from the beginning of time, though to an extremely small extent.

Although the amounts of radioactive materials seem so small it was recognized over 60 years ago that owing to the large energy released per atomic disintegration, they were sufficient to provide major sources of heat in the earth's crust, amounting to about 6×10^{-6} cal/gm. of rock per year on the average. The total heat production is very large. A simple calculation shows that, making reasonable assumptions, the radioactivity of the earth amounts in all to a heat production equivalent to 32 million megawatts. This may be compared to Great Britain's modest nuclear power programme of about 5,000 megawatts. The energy liberated by radioactivity beneath the surface of this country may be greater than electrical power utilized on the surface. It is interesting, too, that we observe radiation damage to rocks just as we do in the materials of nuclear reactors. The so-called 'pleochroic haloes' are due to alpha particle damage in the minerals biotite and zircon, and it has been calculated that the radiation dose produced by thorium and uranium during geologic time is comparable to that which produces radiation damage effects in the components of nuclear reactors.

These studies of heat flow in the earth's crust under continents and oceans have become important branches of geophysics, for this heat flow is one or two orders of magnitude higher than the more obvious release of energy in earthquakes and volcanoes. Differences in heat accumulation due to radioactivity may be responsible for major geological processes as, for example, in mountain building, and it may well be that natural radioactivity has played a major rôle in the great convexion currents in the earth's crust which has moved continents, transformed climates and moulded the face of the earth to its present forms. If I had to guess how radioactivity had caused most havoc among human beings I should say most probably by earth movements, volcanic eruptions and analogous geophysical phenomena.

The radioactivity of soil derived from rocks gives rise to a flux of nuclear radiation from all land surface which is now known to vary from place to place by orders of magnitude. Both igneous and sedimentary rocks vary in radioactive content and hence give rise to very varying amounts of radiation above them. In general, the beta-ray dose to humans on the earth's surface is negligible and it is the penetrating gamma rays that interest us most. Typical estimates of the dose-rates over limestone may be 20 milli-rad/year, while over a granite area it may be perhaps 150 milli-rad/year. The mean value in this country is about 50 milli-rad/year. It is found that much higher radiation fields exist in some special districts. For instance, in monazite areas in the states of Rio de Janeiro and Espirito Santo, Brazil, a population of 30,000 people is estimated to live in radiation fields of 500 to 1,000 milli-rad/year. In other volcanic intrusive areas in Brazil peak values of 12,000 milli-rad/year have been recorded. This is 100 times greater than normally observed in this country. In large areas of France, containing some sixth of the French population, values are quoted as 180 to 350 milli-rad/year, while in Kerala and Madras states in India values of 1,300 milli-rad/year are recorded, ranging up to the highest values of the order of 4,000 milli-rad/year.

We see, therefore, that there are large differences in the natural gamma rays over the land surfaces of the earth. The significance of these differences in dose-rate could be exaggerated by the possibility that food grown in these districts may also be more radioactive. The same may hold true occasionally for drinking water, though strangely enough we have found a reverse situation in many instances, the waters from radioactive areas in this country tending to be low in activity.

The gamma dose-rate inside buildings is generally different from the value out-of-doors, being increased by the radioactive content of the building (bricks were early shown to be active) and decreased by the shielding effect of the walls. Some concretes incorporating shale give unusually high values of dose-rates and also some fibre board materials used in modern house construction. The relatively high gamma-ray doses inside granite houses are well known. Let us hasten to add that no biological effects of these radiations have been demonstrated.

A small increase in dose-rate may be produced by the accumulation as a result of poor ventilation in buildings of natural radioactive gases radon 222 and radon 220, produced from radium. Industrial atmospheres are usually more highly charged with radon than those of country districts. It is also interesting that air below the surface in the interstices of soil often contains perhaps 1,000 times the concentration of radon to be found in the free air above, and closed spaces such as caves have been known for many years to have high radon content derived from the gas released in the decay of radium and diffusing into the limited volume. This radon in soil delivers appreciable doses to the roots of plants, particularly if there are air volumes near them and must have been of significance as a constituent of the radiation dose given to primitive organisms emerging from the sea on to land. The estimation of the mean dose to a human population exposed to natural gamma rays is not at all easy and many more measurements are needed. Thus insufficient measurements have been made to obtain a reliable estimate of the mean dose-rate to the world's population from these natural environmental gamma radiations, but a reasonable guess would be some 80 milli-rad/year in air, or perhaps 50 milli-rad/year to the gonads or bone.

A second major component of irradiation of human beings arises from cosmic rays, concerning which so much has been learned recently by space exploratory vehicles. At sea level we are irradiated chiefly by high energy muons. Galactic cosmic rays consist mostly of protons, hydrogen nuclei. A swift wind of hydrogen also blows continuously through the solar system, emanating from the sun so that many energetic particles beat down on our planet. Observed cosmic radiation increases as we rise above the earth's surface and so emerge from the shielding influence of our atmosphere which thus helps make life possible by acting as a shielding material as well as a respiratory medium. A rise of 10,000 ft above sea level will increase the intensity of cosmic rays some three times. The intensity of these radiations at 70,000 ft, the proposed level of future supersonic aircraft, is such as to raise some concern for crews continually at such heights, particularly as we know that during so-called 'solar flares' large increases of intensity can occur, even if for short times only. The intensity seems unlikely to be of importance for the individual passenger in the normal high flying aircraft, but for space travel may prove a real difficulty. The existence of 'belts' of radiation above the earth's surface, yielding hundreds of rad per hour, certainly may limit the possible or probable routes of egress for space-craft. Cosmic radiation varies in a complex way with latitude and longitude, but the details of these very interest-ing patterns need not concern us here. In this country at sea level cosmic rays furnish about one-third of our natural radiation dose.

Having looked at the solid earth and upper atmosphere we naturally ask what is the natural radioactive content of the oceans, lakes and rivers? In general, the uranium, thorium, or radium content of sea-water is perhaps a hundred times less than that of soils, but again the activity is variable from ocean to ocean and at different depths. The important radioactivity is that of potassium 40. In bulk, however, other activities are still considerable. The oceans, for instance, contain about 400 tons of radium, about 10^9 curies, but its concentration is very low except in some interesting oceanic sediments. The fascinating and important problem of oceanic circulations, both vertical and horizontal, and the consequent movements of activity cannot detain us, though of obvious interest in relation to possible waste disposal.

Nearer to our everyday practical problems are questions of the radioactivity of surface and particularly drinking waters. It has been known since 1904 that natural waters and in particular spa waters contained radium and also radon gas in relatively high concentrations. Recently my colleagues and I have measured about 100 drinking waters used in the United Kingdom by fair-sized populations and find very variable amounts of radioactivity in them. Similar results of measurements in the United States now give a fairly clear overall picture of the situation, but very large local variations are observed. The highest activities in drinking waters are in spa waters and are due largely to radon, though appreciable radium may occur. Next in order of decreasing activity come waters from boreholes in geological strata other than chalk, followed by waters from boreholes in chalk and surprisingly last, surface waters from rivers, lakes and reservoirs even though derived from areas of precambrian or granitic rock formations. The latter often contain little suspended matter and this is the cause of their low activity. If we assume a daily intake of 2·5 litres of water per head of population, the daily intake of long-lived activity from drinking water may vary by a factor of 500 : 1 from place to place, and amounts roughly to 0·01 μμc to 60 μμc. The radon intake may easily reach 10,000 μμc.

During recent years we have studied the radioactivity of many hundreds of food samples and find again a very wide range of natural radioactivity, largely radium and its products. The ratio of most active to least active foods amounts to 20,000 : 1. In general, fruits and vegetables have very low natural activity with meat and milk slightly higher. The most active type of food met with in bulk is cereals, but the radioactivity of Brazil nuts is most surprising and forty times higher still. About 1 oz of nuts contains as much radium and thorium as the entire skeleton and soft tissues of a normal adult. Most of us ingest perhaps 70 per cent of our daily ration of natural radioactivity in cereals and related foods. In general, the intake of natural radioactivity in this country from foods is an order of magnitude greater than from waters, but this generalization must be treated with caution. It is not so, for example, in some American or even British local populations.

When we examine the air and its radioactivity we meet much complexity. The radon content of air varies widely from place to place and from day to day. On dull foggy days in cities the content tends to be high, while it is usually very low on clear days in the country or at sea. The content of radon over a strongly emanating soil has a well-marked diurnal rhythm, being low at midday and high in the early hours of the morning. It varies with barometric pressure and changes of pressure and with the wind direction.

One of the most interesting developments of the last few years in this field has been the discovery of a natural 'fall-out' cycle. Radon diffuses from the surface of the earth into the upper air at an average rate of about 1 atom per square centimetre of the earth's surface every two seconds, yet this apparently minute leakage has fascinating and observable effects in the biosphere. Following its emergence into the atmosphere the daughter products of radon attach themselves to aerosols and dust particles, continuing to diffuse upwards but decreasing in concentration with height. The polonium-lead-bismuth 214 transforms to a second series of lead-bismuth-polonium 210 which are 'washed out' in rain and thus brought back to earth. We have found that the natural alpha activity of grass is often proportional to rainfall, the deposition being on the average about 1 atom per square centimetre every four seconds. Polonium 210 may then be ingested along with grass by sheep and may be found in very appreciable quantities in their kidneys, to which it gives easily measurable doses of radiation. It is scarcely surprising that we have recently found that polonium 210 is the chief alpha-emitting natural radioactive material in human soft tissues and we estimate that it delivers doses of perhaps 2 to 10 milli-rem/year to human gonads. This finding is highlighted by a fascinating recent discovery that the bones (and we suspect the soft tissues) of some Eskimos and Laplanders have an alpha activity due to polonium 210 perhaps fifty times that normally observed in this country. This arises from the continuous deposition of polonium 210 on lichens which are the chief food of reindeer and caribou, which store it in their soft tissues. These animals are in their turn eaten by Laplanders and Eskimos. This soft tissue 'food chain' may prove as important genetically as that in bone, which has been studied for so long. How pertinent were Rutherford's words written in *Harper's Magazine* for February 1905: 'Every falling raindrop and snowflake carries some of this radioactive matter to the earth, while every leaf and blade of grass is covered with an invisible film of radioactive material'. Please note that these words were written 40 years before the first atomic explosion.

We see, therefore, that we all have been and are subjected to ionizing radiations from our surroundings, food and drink, and even from the air we breathe. In addition, we are exposed to many other natural radioactive substances. A luminous timepiece may contain 2 or 3 million $\mu\mu$c of radium; an incandescent gas mantle is almost pure thorium dioxide with a specific activity such that 1 mgm represents more radioactivity than the usual content of the human body. When I think of my boyhood and the proximity of gas mantles in closed rooms I have sometimes wondered how much radioactivity was ingested by my generation in the form of flakes and fragments of highly active thorium dioxide. The amount of thoron in the air was also unknown. Automatic lighter flints, powders for polishing and cleaning and certain dental fillings have been found to have relatively high activity. Uranium, I am told, was used to colour artificial teeth to make them look natural; all crockery, pottery and sanitary earthenware have measurable activities. Paper glazes often have measurable activity and it is relieving in a mood of perversity to measure the radioactivity of an official report on the dangers of nuclear and allied radiations! An almost untouched field of research lies in the study of the tissues of various animal species. We have measured a few and find that ox bone may be 20 or 30 times more active than human bones, and so may certain sheep. Camel bone has, I believe, the highest activity yet observed in bone, but we have not yet tried reindeer. Though we have few data, man seems to be among the less radioactive species!

Many measurements have been made during the last few years of the natural radioactivity of human tissues and the outlines of the picture are gradually being filled in. Radium 226 is always present in human bone and so, as we have seen, are its breakdown products, though perhaps half of the resulting radon diffuses from the bone and escapes in the breath, thus reducing the amounts of the later members of the series. Thorium 228 is also present, but probably gets into the body via its parent radium 228, since the body cannot distinguish between the two isotopes of radium 226 and 228. It seems that our skeletons do not get more active as we grow older and, indeed, fœtal bones show as high a specific activity as adult bone per gram of material. Perhaps this is not surprising since their materials are derived from adult maternal tissues. We still need many more observations on children, particularly in the 1 to 5 year age group. Small quantities of carbon 14, tritium and potassium 40 make up our normal radioactive content and did so long before nuclear explosions. In general, the main natural activity of soft tissues is potassium 40 supplemented by the alpha-emitter polonium 210, but in the lungs we may find traces of other materials, particularly insoluble particles bearing nuclides such as thorium 232, perhaps uranium 238 and very small quantities of plutonium 239. Industrial workers exposed to radium and uranium may show greatly increased radium activity in bone and, of course, may consequently develop bone sarcomas, but a hundredfold increase of radium in bone may be accompanied by only a threefold increase of activity in soft tissues.

The daily intake of radioactivity by normal people may reach an appreciable fraction of their whole-body burden, but most of this activity is excreted in fæces so that our activity does not increase indefinitely but quickly reaches equilibrium.

We have, therefore, a picture of a naturally radioactive human environment, often of much higher specific activity than our bodies, leading to complex cycles of metabolism, intake and excretion. At the same time we receive radiation from the ground, the soil, the buildings and ourselves. We are irradiated at all times by an intensity of natural radiation which would cause an ionizing event in each of the cells of our body on an average once every two or three days.

Is all this natural radiation and radioactivity of any significance to our health and has it played any part in biological evolution? We cannot answer these questions and, indeed, one has the feeling of fumbling not for answers, but for slightly intelligent questions, namely, questions having any chance of being even partially answered.

In a very speculative mood a case could certainly be made that radioactivity and its associated radiations have been of significance in a variety of ways during evolution. Of recent years there has been much renewed discussion of the 'origin of life' or at least, of the origin of materials required by very simple organisms. The original atmosphere of our planet was probably reducing rather than oxidizing and perhaps consisted of methane, ammonia, water and hydrogen. It was thought that important organic compounds could arise under the action of ultra-violet light or electric discharges on such an atmosphere. Recently it has been shown experimentally that a few natural amino-acids can, indeed, be produced in such conditions, and since it is difficult to visualize a primeval form of life not centred around proteins these findings open exciting possibilities. Investigation is now tending to be centred on the formation of such biologically important compounds by heat, but the very high ionizing conditions to be found in soils and the well-known significance of ionization in facilitating chemical reactions inevitably raises the question whether natural radioactivity might not have played a part in the formation of the first biocompounds. Nuclear energy may well have been involved in the emergence of life and the suggestion has at least the merit that radioactivity and its accompanying ionization ensures a supply of energy of an effective type at the right place. Perhaps life is also beginning now! We have, at least, less reason to exclude this possibility than we had formerly.

The question might, of course, be asked whether ionizing radiation is necessary to life. It seems improbable, but we have little evidence. Attempts to change the fraction of potassium 40 in living organisms and so their internal dose have given negative results, but it is interesting to ask whether there are any organisms not naturally exposed. Where, in fact, would we expect the lowest radiation?[16] Clearly, not at high altitudes owing to intense cosmic rays; certainly not below ground, unless some less active geological formations are discovered. A man standing above a granite plane surface receives from the granite about half of the radiation which might strike him if he were completely surrounded. If he wishes to escape radiation he should hastily take a boat and row out to sea, when he will receive only cosmic rays plus half the very low radiation from the ocean.

A large fish or whale near the surface of the water may receive perhaps 65 milli-rad/year, and at 100 metres deep only about 30 milli-rad/year, almost entirely due to their own potassium 40. A very small micro-organism at a depth of 100 metres may receive less than 5 milli-rad/year in the ocean. It is, however, in deep fresh water that we should look for the most extreme variation in natural exposure. If an organism is small (a few microns diameter), and lies in deep clear radioactive-free water and stays away from the bottom (since some sediments have high radium con-

tents and may cau e dose-rates up to 500 milli-rad/year) it
could remain remarkably free from radiation (less than
1 milli-rad/year). It would be interesting to find out how
phyto-plankton of 10 microns diameter that seek the deeper
portions of the euphotic zone of clear lakes respond to
their extremely low dose-rate, since only one phyto-
plankton in about 500 would be expected to experience an
ionizing event before it divided.

Such considerations lead on to the significance of radiation
during evolution. The first naive question might be whether
it raised the mutation rate and so provided necessary
flexibility and speeded evolution. Perhaps more important,
we may ask whether radiation has widened the possible
limits of variation, a question closely related to whether
or not the mutations brought about by ionizing radiations
are the same as those occurring naturally by other
mechanisms, the radiation merely increasing their frequency. The answer usually given to this question is that
they are the same, radiation merely raising the frequency
of spontaneous mutation, but I personally have never been
convinced of this. One could so easily imagine how the
drastic impact of ionization might bring about a change of
gene spectrum not possible, or grossly improbable, in gene
mutations produced by changes of temperature, or by the
more selective mutagenesis of specific chemical compounds.
Of course, unusual and pronounced mutations might well
not survive, and it may be argued that such changes have
already been rejected during natural selection, but I feel
we should still leave this question open. We have seen that
the spectrum of mutation in man is too wide to be included
in a single category for estimating meaningful values of

'doubling dose'. The doubling dose for gross chromosome mutations may well differ considerably from that for point mutation. If so, the frequency distribution of hereditary defects resulting from a specific increase in the level of exposure to radiation might not parallel the natural spectrum.

For some years I have felt that the possible effects of natural radiation during the earlier stages of terrestrial evolution should be carefully looked at. The range of radiation rates from deep water to active rock surface is tremendous and the circumstances of emergence of life must have been extremely variable. We know very little of the changes of natural radiation over hundreds of millions of years, and it could be that alterations of magnetic field (known from other evidence to have occurred) might have affected solar particle flux. It has been suggested that the geologically sudden disappearance of a main group of reptiles from the land, sea and air about 300 million years ago was a possible example of the reduction of population due to high radiation flux! The radiation poured into the germ plasm of some phyla during 200 million years is very large and particularly if asexual reproduction occurs, one cannot help wondering how any deleterious effects were eliminated. Unicellular organisms, multiplying by binary fission, cannot help transmitting cytoplasmic organization as well as genetic code from parent to progeny. Are there mechanisms of deletion of which we are totally unaware? Is there removal of radiation effects at syngamy in simple organisms? We ask, too, what is the rôle of cytoplasmic change?

Perhaps a mere physicist should not pursue such speculations, but I raise the questions here not only because of their intrinsic interest but also to add the remark that I am continually reminded of the delight of Rock Carling in such discussion. We talked of such topics many times and the conversations, I am sure, formed the background of his famous (some thought infamous) question as to whether one mutation which results in an Aristotle, a Leonardo, a Newton, a Gauss, a Pasteur, an Einstein might outweigh ninety-nine that lead to mental defectives.[3]

Is there any evidence that natural radiation has influenced the incidence of any disease such as leukæmia or bone sarcoma? There is a philosophy that by doubling or even trebling the radiation dose from natural background, the effects should not be demonstrable. Certain localized areas support sizeable populations with success, yet have a natural background up by a factor of 10 or even 30 on that observed in this country. It has been suggested *inter alia* that all aging is due to natural radiation background. My only comment would be that I know of no evidence. With respect to leukæmia, it has been thought from several lines of argument (such as the study of atomic bomb survivors, patients suffering from ankylosing spondylitis, radiologists, thymic enlargement) that the probability of inducing leukæmia per individual per rad per year is 1 to 2 per million. This has led to estimates that 10 to 20 per cent of observed leukæmia may be due to background radiation. There is, however, evidence against the basic assumptions made in such calculations, namely, that there is a linear relation of dose to leukæmic effect irrespective of such factors as time since irradiation, age at irradiation, dose-rate. Moreover, variations of incidence of the disease with time following irradiation has now been demonstrated.

A survey of leukæmia in Scotland, in some regions of higher natural backgrounds, by Court-Brown, Spiers and collaborators showed that over an 18-year period the death rate from leukæmia was nearly 50 per cent more than the national average for Scotland, yet the difference in radiation level was 20 per cent or less. Thus it seems we are driven to conclude that we have either under-estimated the effect of background by 100 or more, or that it is much less important than other factors. The last view seems more probable. Attempts to prove higher incidence of leukæmia in Cornwall, where there are high backgrounds, have also proved inconclusive.

A survey of the incidence of congenital malformations in different regions has suggested that higher incidences are associated with geographical areas with high background radiation, and another survey has suggested relation with geomagnetic latitude and hence cosmic rays, but both are quite unconvincing. It is difficult to prove that natural radiation is, in fact, the direct influencing factor. There is no evidence that natural radiation influences the cancer rate in man and this is not surprising since its intensity is rarely one-hundredth of the lowest dose-rate so far shown to induce malignant disease in man or animals.

Measurements made over a wide area indicated 70 to 175 milli-rad/year as the external environmental range of dose-rates of populated areas of the United States, with lower dose-rates prevailing in the more populated eastern and mid-western states.[17] An examination of the frequency of bone sarcoma has been made in the United States in relation to low level radiation exposure. Primary bone tumours were estimated to cause 2,000 deaths a year, decreasing slightly from 1949 to 1955. There is a peak of incidence at about 20 years of age. The analysis of mortality data for bone tumours over a period of seven years involving 14,000 deaths in $1 \cdot 16 \times 10^9$ man-years fails to show any increase in the frequency of the disease in the regions of highest radiation exposure. Indeed, the contrary situation appeared to prevail. These facts are also in accord with earlier observation.

In Great Britain, following investigations of radioactivity of food and water and the corresponding variations of daily intake of radium 226, Turner investigated the correlation between the incidence of a number of sites of cancer and the radioactivity of drinking water. The data do not provide any evidence of any association between cancer mortality rates (i.e. carcinoma of the breast, uterus, trachea, lung, bronchus, stomach or leukæmia) and the natural radio-activity of the drinking water. Indeed, the areas of Wales which show surplus mortality from gastric cancer possess drinking waters with low content of activity. There is, I think, less enthusiasm than there was a few years ago for geographical studies on possible genetic effects of back-ground radiation. On the physical side it has been abun-dantly demonstrated that the task of finding accurately the mean dose to a human population is extremely difficult. The high radioactivity and, therefore, radiation dose of some districts tends to occur in very localized areas and integration over the whole moving population is uncertain. Perhaps, however, the main difficulties arise in the genetic field. We have seen how complex the influence of social structure may be, involving mating habits, age structure, religion, race, even social services, which may be bringing about large changes in the genetic structure of these populations at the same time as we are looking for possibly much smaller ones. In a survey published by the World Health Organization in 1959[18] detailed study was made of the type of information needed, the statistical problems involved and the many other factors which require to be taken into account in such studies. It seems improbable that we are going to get information quickly, and all I would be prepared to say is that present observations suggest that factors other than radiation are of more importance in defining geopathology. Nevertheless, I still think this is a fascinating subject, well worth pursuing even in connection with natural radiation.

Chapter 4

ARTIFICIAL RADIOACTIVITY

We will now review briefly[6, 7, 19] the radiation that man has recently added to his environment by the explosion of nuclear devices and by other less spectacular but possibly more important means, as for example by the increasing medical use of X rays. There is an enormous but uneven literature on this subject and the cynic might well maintain that so far as 'fall-out' is concerned, the experts are well buried beneath mountains of often trivial numerical data. Numbers are poured upon us but comprehension is another matter.

Nuclear weapons differ in their construction and size and may be detonated in a number of ways and in different media; under water, on or just above land or in the air. Underground explosions should lead to little distribution and deposition of radioactive material, though care must be taken that radioactive gases do not escape from fissures and that the fission products from the explosion do not contaminate underground sources of water supplies. The explosions of most interest, namely, those in the air above ground, give rise to a very large quantity of radioactive material much of which is carried into the upper atmosphere where rainfall does not occur and the rate of vertical diffusion is much slower than in the lower so-called 'troposphere'. This is particularly true of explosions well above the surface of the earth. The height to which the material rises depends upon the size and the characteristics of the bomb, but a very large number of radioactive materials are formed. The larger particles produced in the explosion fall to the earth relatively close to the site of explosion, but a considerable fraction of the activity is carried in or on fine dust particles which remain airborne for long enough to diffuse widely throughout the upper atmosphere and affect large areas of the earth's surface. They tend to be carried down to the earth at about the latitude of their production. The total activity decreases with time, and as the initial mixture contained many materials of different half-lives, the composition of the debris changes with time, the longer-lived components eventually predominating. We need consider only those materials produced in sufficient amount and having chemical and physical properties likely to make them of biological or medical significance. During the first few days after an explosion iodine constitutes an important part of the radioactive material, followed in sequence of significance by zirconium, niobium, cerium and many others, but after a few months caesium 137 and particularly strontium 90 assume prime importance.

The radioactive products may enter the body in a variety of ways, for example, by inhalation or following deposition on vegetables eaten by humans or transference to humans via animals used as human food. They may fall into drinking water supplies and thence again be ingested by humans. In general, the concentrations of material in the air are low and inhalation is not an important general hazard. It is possible to detect and measure in normal human lungs plutonium 239 derived from explosions, but this is a technical *tour de force* rather than of practical interest. In spite of the low atmospheric concentration the continuous deposition of caesium 137 on to the ground gives rise to external irradiation analogous to the natural gamma rays from the earth. The caesium will also be taken up by humans from milk, meat and other foods. The particular importance of strontium 90 arises from a curious chain of circumstances. It is produced in large quantities in the initial fission processes of a nuclear explosion and is effectively carried to the earth's surface in the great atmospheric circulations of cold polar air whose movement gives rise to a maximum deposition of strontium 90 in spring and early summer. The deposition is chiefly via rain. Once deposited, strontium 90, with its long half-life of 25 years, remains near the surface and is ingested by grazing cattle. Being chemically analogous to calcium, the radioactivity is fairly efficiently conveyed to the cow's milk, which we then use as the sole diet of the most sensitive part of the population, infants engaged in growing new bones and requiring good supplies of calcium. Moreover, the strontium is concentrated in bone of relatively small volume and hence delivers a large radiation dose.

To return to the overall picture, the relative importance of internal and external irradiation by fission products varies from place to place on the earth's surface. In general, deposition is greatest in medium northern latitudes at about 50°N, a kind of poetic justice since Powers letting off bombs tend to reside at about this latitude. The fall-out is less in equatorial or polar regions, though the pattern and the time-scale of deposition depends to some extent on the latitude at which the nuclear device was exploded. In general, the deposition of strontium 90 is roughly proportional at a given place to its rainfall.

The radiation dose-rate at any moment depends both on the total of a given material which has been deposited over the whole testing period, and also on the rate of deposition, chiefly in the months immediately preceding. The former factor tends to be of major importance for strontium 90 and the latter for caesium 137. The amount taken up by a given population depends, too, on the pattern of its diet, for example, what fraction of its calcium it derives from milk, and whether fish plays an important rôle. The circumstances are varied and lead to surprising local differences.

Immediately following nuclear explosions a very important component of fall-out is iodine 131. It is found particularly in milk and is concentrated in the thyroid gland of those ingesting it. It stays in that gland on an average for perhaps ten days. Careful studies have been made of the uptake by humans of iodine from fall-out and particularly of the dose given to small children's thyroids. Following a short period of testing we observe a rise and fall of concentration in milk, and therefore of radiation dose-rate to the thyroid gland as the concentration in milk changes over a few weeks. The estimated doses in this country to thyroids have been small (perhaps not more than a quarter of background radiation). The significance of these short-period rises of radioactivity in milk can easily be misunderstood. If we are concerned with possible cancer of the thyroid in perhaps 20 years time, the important radiation parameter is the total dose integrated over a long period. We must then average observed concentrations of iodine in milk and resulting dose-rates over perhaps a year and not pay too much attention to relatively high instantaneous peaks of activity except in so far as they affect the total amount of radiation received. If we are worried about an effect which is dependent on dose-rate, then of course these peaks might be more significant. The decision by the Medical Research Council to limit the allowed concentration of iodine 131 to 200 pc/litre in milk averaged over a period of one year, still represents in my view a very conservative approach.

The isotope whose dangers have received most consideration is probably strontium 90, a beta ray emitter of 25 years half-life, chemically analogous to calcium and therefore with a similar (but fortunately not exactly identical) metabolism. There is a fairly constant relative discrimination between the two elements in their transfer from human diet to human bone, the ratio in plasma or in human bone being approximately one-quarter of the mean ratio of strontium to calcium in the total diet. This empirically determined ratio is of great practical importance.

Roots of plants do not, in general, discriminate in uptake of calcium and strontium from culture solutions or normal soil water, so that vegetable foodstuffs tend to have the same ratio as the soils in which they grow. In mammals some physiological barriers discriminate. The main route of excretion of strontium is via the urine and it is excreted preferentially by the kidneys as compared with calcium. There is also a substantial discrimination factor at the placental barrier. Admirable studies of the metabolism of strontium in man have been made by Loutit and his colleagues.[11]

The main problems arise with children. Since the intake of strontium 90 might be an important social problem, there has been careful monitoring of foodstuffs and waters in this country for a number of years. Since 1958 the Agricultural Research Council[20] has been responsible for measurements of the degree of contamination of foods which provide substantial amounts of calcium to the national diet. For administrative purposes England is divided into ten regions, which with Scotland and Northern Ireland make up twelve zones. The milk of the zones is sampled at source according to a statistical plan and, in all, effectively 40 per cent of the country's production is measured. Cheese is also sampled as well as vegetable sources of calcium such as cereals, leaf and root vegetables. Drinking water is also sampled and estimates of mean intake by the population are made. Incidentally, it may be said that, in general, the pattern of activity due to strontium 90 in drinking water is the exact opposite of the natural activity, namely, high values in surface waters and virtual absence from deep wells.

Simultaneously with the studies of human foodstuffs measurements are made of human bones. Bones cannot, of course, be collected on a statistical plan, but depend on the chances of fate and the good offices of pathologists. There is very fortunately difficulty in obtaining data concerning young children whose growth rate is high but whose mortality is low. The concentration of strontium 90 in bone of infants is low, which is not surprising for they have after all derived nutrients from adult maternal plasma which is also low. We remember the analogous situation with the radium content of bone. There has been a rise of concentration of strontium 90 over the years in adult bone.[6] The maximum specific activity of bone so far observed is in children between 1 to 2 years of age, when it rises to some ten times the final value in adult bone. Detailed studies of population cohorts enable estimates to be made of strontium metabolism taking into account not only growth but also accompanying turnover of existing bone. The maximum concentration values observed in children are about 3 μμc of strontium 90 per gm calcium, but only about 0·2 μμc/gm calcium in adults. The Medical Research Council considered that the maximum permissible concentration of strontium 90 in bone averaged over the whole population should not exceed 67 μμc/gm, the maximum for any individual member of the population being set at 200 μμc/gm calcium. The corresponding dose-rates to bone are 180 and 540 milli-rem/year and to bone marrow 60 and 180 milli-rem/year respectively. The average dose-rate from natural radiation is about 130 milli-rem/year. Thus the allowed added rates in this country are of the order of natural background and we have seen that no effect has been demonstrable on bone tumour incidence at these levels, though the incidence of the disease is very low and consequently statistics are too poor to demonstrate any but gross percentage effects.

Owing to the slow deposition from the upper atmosphere and the time taken for the material to pass through the 'food chain' there is a considerable time lag between a particular series of nuclear explosions and the time at which the bones even of children reach their maximum activity. We have to try to anticipate the course of events and, if administrative action is required, then it may have to be taken early in any rising activity. Optimists and pessimists find it difficult to agree when that action should be taken, or if it should be taken at all! It would be easy to take drastic administrative action in respect of milk supplies which could do more harm than good. We have also to remember that in areas of low agricultural productivity and high rainfall, higher values of strontium 90 in milk can occur than in other regions. Milk from such sites reaches concentrations four times higher than the average.

The situation after a long and important series of nuclear explosions such as has occurred recently needs very careful watching.[20, 21, 22] The effects of the tests during 1961 and 1962 are only now becoming fully apparent. Fortunately, the best estimates suggest that the mean level of strontium 90 in the bones of young children in the population of any large region of this country is not expected to reach 10 $\mu\mu$c/gm calcium, giving about 30 milli-rem/year. The country-wide averages are not expected to be more than 7 $\mu\mu$c strontium 90 per gram calcium, giving about 20 milli-rem/year. These are quite within the allowed limits, and it will be remembered that so far we have no evidence of bone tumour production at five times these levels of natural activity.

A second isotope of strontium, strontium 89, owing to its short half-life only gives a significant tissue dose during the year following weapons trials and the dose was probably not greater on the average than 25 milli-rem/year.

We will now consider caesium 137. This long-lived nuclide has higher activities than strontium 90 in fall-out, but is held in soil in forms largely inaccessible to plants and its uptake is more markedly influenced by the rate of fall-out. It is an alkali metal like potassium and sodium, being fairly freely absorbed in the intestinal tract and remaining in the body for an average of some three months with considerable individual variation. It is widely distributed throughout the body but found particularly in muscle. Its chief dietary sources are meat and milk, about half from the latter in a typical western diet.

The external radiation due to caesium 137 is estimated at about 1·5 milli-rad/year or about 1 per cent of natural radiation and the mean dose-rate due to soft tissue caesium 137 is also about 1·5 milli-rad/year. These values, however, estimated in 1958, are now probably low by a factor of perhaps two.

One of the most controversial isotopes has been carbon 14. As we have indicated, it is produced naturally as well as artificially. It is rapidly oxidized to carbon dioxide and so enters the natural carbon cycle. As the result of biological processes and the circulation of the oceans, the carbon contained in the atmosphere, in living matter and in the oceans, changes its distribution at a rate which is rapid on a geological time-scale, but reasonably short compared to the long mean life of carbon 14. The annual dose to the whole body due to natural carbon 14 is small and about 1 milli-rad. The possible genetic significance of carbon 14 lies in the fact that carbon atoms make up about 37 per cent of DNA. Hence if a carbon atom is incorporated in a DNA molecule, this molecule may be damaged not only by the ionizing beta particles emitted and the recoiling nucleus, but also by the transmutation of carbon 14 to nitrogen 14 in the process. In this way a viable gene mutation might be produced.

There is some little doubt as to the amount of this material so far produced in nuclear explosions, but up to the end of 1958 it was about 13×10^{27} atoms. In 1959 there was considerably more artificial carbon 14 in the northern hemisphere than in the southern. The mean stratospheric residence time is about five years. It is estimated that the total added dose to gonads due to material released up to 1959 would be about 120 milli-rads but, of course, delivered over thousands of years. This value is to be compared to the total gonad dose due to fall-out from fission products which is estimated to be about 25 milli-rad for the 30 years commencing 1954 with little after that. The gonad dose from natural background would be about 3,000 milli-rad per 30-year period.

Chapter 5

IONIZING RADIATION
OF MISCELLANEOUS ORIGIN

There are a number of other uses of ionizing radiations which contribute small doses to the general population.[5, 6] For example, X-ray fluoroscopy may be used for shoe fitting. Suffice it that this makes only a very small total contribution to the irradiation of the population and, thanks to acceptance by the trade of some control, it is improbable that it is of any general consequence. Obviously care is needed on behalf of operators of equipment and over-enthusiastic children.

The use of luminous clocks and watches may contribute a genetic dose of 1 milli-rad/year to the general public, but the mean radioactive content of these dials seems to be decreasing and the substitution of other isotopes such as tritium for radium has probably improved the situation. The main problems are, again, in the protection of workers in the industry. Television equipment is negligible as a general source of ionizing radiation, but could give significant doses in certain special circumstances to development and maintenance engineers.

The dose received during occupational exposure in this country, chiefly from industrial radiography and the multifarious uses of radioisotopes, is certainly in need of continual surveillance. As a contribution to the genetic dose to the population it is not large, probably not more than a quarter per cent of the natural background, but here again the main problem is the possible somatic damage to a small number of individuals accidentally exposed to doses of the order of a few rad. This is one of the most worrying aspects of protective measures and each year a few cases of exposures to doses up to hundreds of rad are reported. Elaborate safety codes are available, but this is primarily a problem of education and individual responsibility.

In the United Kingdom Atomic Energy Authority itself the record is good not only so far as industrial accidents are concerned but also radiation exposure. The latest Report of the Authority (Tenth Report, 1963 to 1964)[23] records that the number of employees classified as radiation workers is about 20,000 and that the maximum permissible whole-body dose (3 rems in 13 weeks) was exceeded on only four occasions and on one occasion due to inhalation of tritium. The mean dose was very small. Steps were taken in each case to adjust subsequent exposure and ensure that long-term dose limits were not exceeded. The lost-time frequency rate is about 1 per 100,000 man-hours worked.

It is interesting that in consigning 102,000 packages of radioactive materials in the previous year (1962 to 1963) no incidents involving radioactive hazard to the public or employees of transport undertakings occurred, but two vehicles carrying radioactive materials were involved in serious traffic accidents!

There are tremendous local and technical problems in the handling and disposal of radioactive wastes, but so far as the general public is concerned the dose given is extremely small as may be seen from an excellent report.[24] The dose at the moment is quite negligible genetically.

We have already mentioned that industrial radiography and some special techniques such as X-ray crystallography constitute a main industrial hazard from X rays. They are relatively well understood and safety measures are available, but there are regions of industrial activity in which the chief problems are fundamental ignorance and extreme technical difficulty as, for instance, in the handling of plutonium in large quantities. The questions of 'enriched fuels' may become of great importance in the future and fundamental research into the problems of particulate retention in lungs and the effects of localized alpha emitters is urgently needed.

There can be no doubt that much the largest man-made contribution to irradiation of the population at the present time is that associated with the medical use of X rays in diagnostic radiology. Therapeutic radiology adds only a small contribution by the irradiation of patients often with advanced malignant disease, elderly and of low fertility, so that its contribution to genetic dose is low. However, much of the contribution to genetic dose from radiotherapy arises from the treatment of non-malignant disease and could be substantially reduced.

In 1955 the number of persons undergoing X-ray examinations within the National Health Service in this country was 12.2 million and possibly in the whole population some 18 million. A limited survey in the following year indicated a genetic dose to the population of 22 millirad/year. In view of these findings, at the request of the Medical Research Council, a second more widely-spread investigation was made, and in 1960 a Report on Radiological Hazards to Patients was published by a Committee under the chairmanship of Lord Adrian.[13] As the result of this comprehensive national survey the total annual genetic dose from medical radiology in 1957 was shown to be 19.3 milli-rem per person, 14.1 milli-rem per person from diagnostic radiology and 5.2 milli-rem from radiotherapy. We note that the total dose is some 15 to 20 per cent of natural background and constitutes the largest man-made contribution to the irradiation of the population. In other countries the figures are often higher, as may be seen from the very comprehensive data given in the second report of the United Nations Scientific Committee on the Effects of Atomic Radiation.[7] For example, the corresponding annual genetic doses are 27.5 milli-rad/year in Denmark, 58.2 in France, 43.4 in Italy, 39 in Japan and 37 in Sweden. From the United States genetic doses as high as 140 milli-rad/year have been reported and 50 milli-rad/year may be regarded as the minimum. In this country the radiotherapy of non-malignant conditions contributed 4.5 milli-rad, the radiotherapy of malignant conditions 0.5 milli-rad, the medical use of radioactive isotopes 0.18 milli-rad and mass miniature and dental radiography each added the low value of 0.01 milli-rad.

There are, however, some interesting points about the results. Five types of diagnostic examination contribute over 80 per cent of the total genetic dose in this country, namely, obstetric and abdominal examinations (26 per cent), pyelography (13 per cent), pelvimetry (8 per cent), examination of pelvis, lumbar spine and lumbar sacral joint (23 per cent) and hip and upper femur (11 per cent) respectively. The Adrian Committee noted that if greater consideration was given to improvements in diagnostic techniques, particularly careful limitation of beam size and adequate filtration, the dose of 19 milli-rem per person might be reduced to 6 milli-rem or even less with no loss of diagnostic efficiency.

It is not surprising that diagnostic radiology provides the dose. The output of modern X-ray equipment is such that it easily produces at the patient an intensity of radiation 3,000 million times greater than natural radiation and there are obviously good reasons for keeping times of exposure very small. There is no inherent vice in diagnostic radiology, which is necessarily involved in using relatively very powerful beams of X rays on patients and, therefore, in some instances, irradiating their gonads.

Naturally, this finding has given rise to some apprehension, a little research and considerable speculation. Studies of the increasing incidence in diagnosed leukæmia in children in the last 30 years (perhaps by a factor of 2) has led to the conclusion that children who have been X rayed *in utero* are twice as likely to die of malignant disease before their tenth birthday as other children. This is a serious result, but must be seen in proportion. Since at present about one in every 1,200 children in Britain die in this way, it would imply that rather less than one in a thousand of the pre-natal X-ray examinations performed in recent years have led to death from malignant disease before the age of 10. There is, moreover, great difficulty and uncertainty in these investigations. Deaths from leukæmia in this age group even during a period of 10 years are so few that the difference between control and irradiated groups are very small. It may be that if leukæmia is induced in children by diagnostic radiation it is too infrequent to detect with certainty. Nevertheless, it is possible that the capacity of X rays for the production of leukæmia is ten times greater in the fœtus than at any other age, and recently in a large survey of 700,000 children in the United States[25] it was found that the cancer mortality of the X-rayed group was 1.4 times that of the unirradiated. In Denmark, too, there is evidence that diagnostic radiology cannot be neglected as a cause of leukæmia. It would seem wise when possible to avoid or delay diagnostic irradiation of pregnant women and to reduce the dose to the minimum.

In this country, of the children dying of leukæmia and other malignant diseases, over 80 per cent are not irradiated as fœtuses *in utero*, so that for the vast majority this hazard is irrelevant. Most leukæmias in children may be determined before conception so that even of the remaining 20 per cent or so which are irradiated the radiation may be irrelevant. It seems, nevertheless, that in perhaps 5 per cent the radiation may have played a part. While we may be wise to concentrate on studying the 95 per cent or so in which the radiation is not important, the possible production of leukæmia as a result of diagnostic examination of pregnant women is an important question, and fortunately one in which we are able to do something by improved techniques. It must be emphasized that the risk is small.

In all, my own impression is that the man-made radiation which must give rise to most thought in the near future is probably diagnostic radiology. Fortunately we have an overwhelming case for insisting on the usefulness of this type of examination and any attempt to curtail its use could create risks much greater than those we wish to avoid.

Part II

Some social problems in the
control of radiation

Chapter 6

SOME PROBLEMS OF NOMENCLATURE

From a review of facts we turn to wider questions concerning some of the primary concepts involved in the use and control of radiation. Can there be in any real sense a 'safe dose of radiation'?

In the early days of X-ray therapy experience suggested there was a 'threshold' for the production of erythema below which no effect was seen and above which there was an observable reddening of the skin. This 'threshold erythema dose' was the subject of much research and my own early excursions into the radiation field were concerned with trying to find its value in terms of the then new 'r' units.

This concept of 'threshold' became deeply embedded in radiological thought and led quite naturally to the concept of a 'tolerance dose' (in the old nomenclature) below which crudely you were 'safe' and above which unpleasant things would happen.

It was realized that the effects of X rays involved intense spots of localized energy absorption and thence disruption of biological structures, but somehow Nature repaired these micro-events and macroscopically all might still be well. The idea of a working threshold is even now not the foolish concept some would have us believe, and radiotherapy and radiodiagnosis rely in great measure upon its practical validity.

It is, however, when we examine the statistics of rare diseases in large populations or argue about genetics that we begin to be more wary. If in the genetic field biological effect is accurately proportional to dose it is argued that even the smallest dose produces some 'effect' and there is no 'threshold'. There is no 'safe' dose. Of course, a practical threshold could arise because the biological effect was so long delayed in appearance that death of the organism intervened. If there is a 20 year period between irradiation and the appearance of cancer a number of people may have died before the disease manifests itself. The presence or absence of an observed threshold depends upon the patience of the observer, particularly as the delay in appearance of effect may increase as the dose decreases. A Medical Research Council Report[6] summed up this difficult question as follows: 'Any radiation exposure is likely to produce some change in at least a few cells, although the normal process of tissue repair may be adequate to reverse these changes if they are very slight or if they occur at a very low rate. The essential difficulty is to decide whether an apparent threshold is due to a genuine absence of effect at low doses or to a failure to observe the effect owing to the very low frequency with which it is occurring. It might be due to the latter if the frequency with which an effect occurred were directly proportional to the dose received, but would be even more likely to be so if this frequency were proportional to the square of the dose or to some other power'.

'There are great practical difficulties in planning any investigation to decide these issues. The probability of the occurrence of harmful effects following low doses may be so small or the delay in their induction so prolonged as to make it impossible to design a sufficiently extensive study to demonstrate them. This difficulty applies particularly to the investigation of the effects on man of low doses received at a slow rate, like the radiation from the natural background or from artificial sources such as fall-out which give even smaller rates'.

I have always felt that the argument that because at higher values of dose an observed effect is proportional to dose, then at very low doses there is necessarily some 'effect' of dose, however small, is nonsense. The 'exposure dose' consists of a finite number of quanta. The 'effect', namely a 'hit', and the subsequent alteration of a gamete is also 'quantized' in time (because of the finite sensitive life of a unit) and in space. When the 'exposure dose' is very small and the gamete is transient, as the dose-rate decreases there is an increasing probability of a particular gamete escaping altogether. It may be said that the 'absorbed dose' in that gamete is then zero and we have to define 'dose' rather carefully. In a population of gametes, as exposure dose decreases an increasing number escape altogether, and therefore the probability increases that any subsequent fertilization will be the work of 'unirradiated' gametes. The individual has escaped effect; the population may not.

The important difficulty lies in grasping that one is not talking about a relation of 'dose' to 'effect', but the correlation between the very small probability of an ionizing event in a given small region during a given time interval and the even smaller probability of that event emerging as a biologically significant alteration within a given time.

Maybe these considerations should worry a theoretical physicist very little. He is well aware that many of the 'laws of physics' are statistical rules which hold only for very large numbers of events. If one puts the kettle on the fire there is a calculable probability that the water will freeze. Some things never happen in the physical world because they are impossible, others because they are too improbable. These two ways of attaining zero have been badly confused in the genetic argument.

Philosophically, too, the physicist is happier than the biologist in this argument, for Physics is no longer pledged to a scheme of deterministic law. In studying mutations we are thinking of quantum leaps in complex molecules. Living, as I do, on Epsom Downs and therefore not unacquainted with the economic consequences of genetics in species other than man, I turn to Eddington: 'The quantum physicist does not fill the atom with gadgets for directing its future behaviour as the classical physicist would have done; he fills it with gadgets determining the odds on its future behaviour. He studies the arts of the bookmaker not of the trainer'.[26]

You will have observed that I have not answered the question as to whether there is a 'safe dose', but only discussed the difficulties of visualizing and defining the lower limit of risk, but we must now pass to the next question, presuming some risk but not necessarily effect, for all doses greater than zero. This is a strict criterion which would revolutionize the philosophy of industrial hazards generally and if applied rigorously could bring great industries to a standstill on the grounds that no risk to employees was allowed.

The formal definition of effect at very low doses dissolves into small probabilities and indefiniteness. At the upper limit of defined 'safe dose', namely, the so-called 'maximum permissible dose', most people complain that the connotations are not too vague, but much too definite. It seems to resemble too closely Mr. Micawber's financial precipice; on one side all is happiness and light, on the other ruin and destruction.

The old term 'tolerance dose' has fallen into disuse though it had at least the merit of indicating that someone 'tolerated' it. What was not clear was whether this 'someone' was the recipient of the dose or the Protection Committee. The term 'maximum permissible dose' has always seemed to me to be more rigid and rather to imply some omniscient creature sagaciously fixing limits from above. A more accurately descriptive term would, I believe, have been 'maximum permitted dose', indicating clearly an element of arbitrary judgement (which there certainly is) and perhaps fallibility in our present knowledge. The question becomes even more tangled when a certain time of exposure is required to produce an effect. We may be able to withstand a given concentration of a toxic agent for a certain time, but indefinite exposure might be seriously harmful. We may be prepared to tolerate a given level of iodine in milk for a year but not indefinitely. We may see little harm in an even higher value for iodine concentration for a few days but not for a year.

Recently (May 1960) the American Federal Radiation Council, set up to advise the American President, has attempted to introduce the concept of 'radiation protection guides' to avoid some of these difficulties. The 'radiation protection guide', says the report prepared by the Council,[27] 'is the radiation dose which should not be exceeded without careful consideration of the reasons for doing so'. I know that the concept of 'maximum permissible level' and a fixed numerical value is perhaps rigid, but the wording relative to the 'guide' seems not so much a definition of a dose as an acknowledgement of irresponsibility. One cannot help wondering who is going to do the considering and what reasons might be advanced.

I see no answer to this problem of misinterpretation of fixed levels except education of administrators, scientists and general public. The fixing of a 'danger level' is an exercise in administration which involves some arbitrary decisions. It is not entirely or often primarily scientific, though it is sometimes heralded as having a precise scientific basis.

We have a 30 mile an hour speed limit on many roads. No one pretends that a little below 30 miles an hour we are safe or that just above it we are as good as dead, yet the choice of 30 is not entirely arbitrary. It is obvious why the limit is not 3 or 300, but there is an element of arbitrariness about the decision. We can argue as between 30 and 40. Perhaps one of the main purposes of setting a fixed limit is to make a social and psychological separation between those who are careful and mostly obey a rule and those who do not. Perhaps a 'maximum permissible level' is set for much the same reason! There are great risks on the roads at all speeds, even at zero. We wonder whether anyone sat down and calculated how this risk increased with speed and how much risk we ought to take or be allowed to take, and so arrived at the magic number 30.

We are back at the question whether there is a safe dose,

but now in a more intelligent form, namely, 'what is an admissible risk' and 'who fixes it'?

Chapter 7

MAXIMUM PERMISSIBLE LEVELS OF RADIATION

The levels of permitted radiation are, of course, legally the responsibility of the governments of the countries concerned, but in practice they nearly all stem from an International Commission on Radiological Protection (I.C.R.P.), which has an interesting origin.

I will make no attempt to outline the detailed history of protective measures, but note that in 1921 a 'British X-ray and Radium Protection Committee' was formed and issued its first 'recommendations' in the same year. Rock Carling was its final chairman.

From 1921 onwards there has been a steady stream of 'recommendations', 'regulations' and, more recently, legislation. If we confine ourselves to international action we note that 'International Recommendations' were adopted by the Second International Congress of Radiology in 1928 and that the form and scope of these edicts (drawn up by the predecessor of I.C.R.P.) still remained much the same up to the time of a Radiological Congress in 1937. The measures outlined (1937)[28] were designed specifically to protect radiological workers from the 'known effects to be guarded against', namely '(a) injuries to superficial tissues, and (b) changes in the blood and derangement of internal organs, particularly the generative organs'. We note, too, that the evidence then available 'appears to suggest that under satisfactory working conditions, a person in normal health can tolerate exposure to X rays and radium gamma rays to an extent of about 0.2 international röntgen (r) per day or 1 r per week'. The 'tolerance dose' (1 r per week) was ten times that now permitted as a continuing occupational exposure. We would have been thought very odd in those days had we suggested the natural background due to radioactivity in the earth or the 'waters under the earth' as a serious social problem.

An excellent report by Wintz and Rump, published in 1931 by the Health Organization of the League of Nations,[29] was remarkable in a number of ways. It reviewed the history of the 'tolerance dose', estimated in 1925 at one-hundredth of an 'erythema dose' (later converted to 6 r) per month and even more remarkably, estimated doses in absolute energy units (1 röntgen being set equivalent to 85 ergs/gram), thus essentially anticipating the 'rad' by 20 years.

After the Second World War the scene changed. Meeting in London in 1950, the newly-constituted International Commission on Radiological Protection (still a technical Committee of the Radiological Congresses) opens its report[30] in more dramatic fashion: 'Developments in nuclear physics and their practical applications since the last International Congress (1937) have greatly increased the number and scope of potential hazards'. The 'effects to be considered' were widened to include '(1) Superficial injuries; (2) general effects on the body, particularly the blood and blood-forming organs, e.g. production of anæmia and leukæmia; (3) the induction of malignant tumours; (4) other deleterious effects, including cataract, obesity, impaired fertility and reduction of life span; (5) genetic effects'. After some other important preliminaries we note the introduction of the term 'whole-body exposure', for which the 'maximum permissible dose' was reduced to 0.5 röntgens per week. This must be one of the first international appearances of this now hallowed phrase. The text of 1950 goes on to discuss 'critical tissues', 'partial body exposure', and a safety factor of 10 for neutrons, one of the earliest values of Relative Biological Effect ('R.B.E.') or Quality Factor ('Q.F.'). It was very cautious about stating 'maximum permissible exposure' to radioactive isotopes, but did fix fundamental limits for Ra226, Pu239, Sr89, Sr90($+$Y90), natural uranium, Po210, H3 (tritium), C14, Na24, P32, Co60, I131, as well as defining the 'Standard Man'. It is only fair to add that these recommendations owed a very great deal to American and subsequent British and Canadian discussion of these subjects within the new atomic energy organizations in those countries. We owe a great deal to the generous help of our American colleagues in those early days.

The Commission's report of 1950 is the first of the modern International Radiological Protection Recommendations. Rock Carling was chairman of this Commission from 1950 to 1956, and those of us who served under him know how much its very existence as well as the clarity and restraint of its recommendations owed to his perspicacity and quiet humour, coupled with a power of evoking trust from representatives of various nationalities in days when the mental scars of war were very sensitive to the touch.

Following 1950 change of detail has been swift. The International Commission on Radiological Protection (I.C.R.P.), still in association with the Congresses of Radiology, now functions in close liaison with the United Nations and its group of committees and special agencies, as for example the United Nations Scientific Committee on the Effects of Atomic Radiation, World Health Organization, International Labour Office, United Nations Educational Scientific and Cultural Organization and the International Atomic Energy Agency. The reports of I.C.R.P. and its Committees now run to hundreds of complex pages and give maximum permissible levels for some 250 radioactive materials. It is a fair guess that I.C.R.P. is now far more widely known than its parent body, for it has become the acknowledged international authority in the field of radiation hazards. This unbelievably sensible situation has greatly helped radiation safety measures everywhere, for even from the U.S.S.R. and Eastern European countries there has been considerable co-operation and essential agreement with the standards of I.C.R.P. The world owes a debt to Rock Carling for having piloted this enterprise in its early formative years.

Historically the next important landmark in measures concerning radiation hazards was the United Nations Conference in Geneva in 1955 on the Peaceful Uses of Atomic Energy. This Conference released a great deal of technical information and stimulated interest in the development of atomic power throughout the world. It also revealed and emphasized the vast field opening up for the use of radioactive isotopes in industry, agriculture and medicine. Correspondingly it focused sharply the problem of the increasing numbers of people likely to be employed in circumstances leading to exposure to radiation. It raised even higher existing concern about the genetic effects of radiation on whole populations. The realization that many of those employed would be relatively unskilled and uninstructed persons made it necessary to disseminate knowledge of protective measures as rapidly and as widely as possible. Education and control became urgent, particularly as protective measures were often complex and expensive and economics could be expected to gnaw at the foundations of 'safety factors'.

In 1956 for the first time the Recommendations of the International Commission on Radiological Protection defined groups of persons whose radiation levels should be treated differently, namely (a) those occupationally exposed; (b) special groups in the vicinity of 'controlled areas'; and (c) the population at large. For the occupationally exposed the old weekly 'tolerance dose' disappeared in favour of a maximum dose of 3 rem in 13 weeks and, in addition, a rule which virtually limits the annual dose to 5 rem over long periods of time. These numbers still derived from old experience with X rays, modified by modern conditions and techniques.

With respect to radioactive materials, there has always been a second line of argument stemming largely from the observed results of radium ingested accidentally by those preparing luminous dials of instruments, watches and clocks. The pathological changes observed, including the production of bone sarcoma in a number of workers, led many years ago to a stipulation that 0.1 μc of radium be the maximum amount allowed in the human skeleton. This number, suitably modified to take account of the nature of the radiation and its distribution in bone was the basis of many 'maximum permissible levels' for bone-seeking isotopes. Some are unhappy at this particular derivation of safety levels, but historically this was its basis and, happily, we have so far no bone tumours produced by strontium 90 in humans to give us guidance.

The I.C.R.P. Recommendations now set out special concentration limits and doses for some single organs and in particular gonads, bone, skin and thyroid. 'Permissible concentrations' of radioactive materials in air and drinking water may be derived mathematically by calculating the concentrations in those media which would maintain the allowed concentrations in the tissues in question. The sums are easy. The fundamental biophysical and physiological assumptions are the difficulty.

So far we have been thinking of those occupationally exposed. Intermediate groups of persons are allowed smaller doses, but we pass them over and proceed to the questions which arise in dealing with the 'general population'. We have now to remember that many circumstances will be different from those in an occupationally exposed group. We now include pregnant women, children and persons suffering from pathological conditions which might render them more sensitive. There are questions of availability of medical services and continual surveillance. The possibility of individual monitoring for radiation exposure will now rarely arise and those concerned may have different occupational hazards of their own. It is, therefore, usually thought that a lower radiation exposure should apply for large populations than for small occupationally exposed groups. We are dealing with a large number of people and a large scale catastrophe is possible. Nevertheless, this distinction between permissible levels, and presumably risks to different members of the population, raises some fundamental questions of human rights.

At very low dose levels possible genetic hazards are evidently the first consideration and will depend predominantly upon the product of the number of people and the average level of irradiation of genetic significance to which they are exposed. This is, so to speak, the total amount of radiation going into that population.

It is held by I.C.R.P. that the 'genetic dose to the whole population for all sources, additional to natural background, should not exceed 5 rem for 30 years, with the lowest practicable contribution from medical exposure'. It will be noted that this is some thirty times below agreed occupational exposure.

In the 30-year period assumed for each generation the natural radiation dose would in this country be about 3 rem, so that the dose allowed is roughly trebling the background. It will be remembered that very much larger variations than this occur naturally as between different places on the earth's surface. The Commission's recommendation is supported by the Medical Research Council, which in 1956 considered it 'unlikely that any authoritative recommendation would name a figure for a permissible radiation dose to the whole population, added to that received from natural sources, which was more than twice that of the general value from the natural background radiation, in this country an average of 3 r per generation of 30 years'. It is difficult to quote a present contribution due to man-made activity, but an increase of genetic dose by 20 per cent of natural background is a reasonable estimate.

If we turn to criticize the present numerical values of

maximum permissible levels laid down by I.C.R.P. we must remember that it is still only some 10 years since the genetic problems of whole populations have officially assumed a status of serious social importance. The restrictions imposed on genetic dose have so far as I am aware not caused any serious embarrassment here and, though they seem strict in view of the much greater known variations of dose-rate over the surface of the earth (without demonstrable effect), it is probably wise to retain the suggested levels. The build-up of deleterious recessive genes in a population will often require many generations, and we may hope that before much harm, if indeed any, be done, our knowledge of chemical genetics will have enabled us to make considerably better-informed guesses and perhaps take more appropriate action or justified inaction. Our present knowledge of rate of production of mutation per unit dose of radiation at very low doses or dosage-rates is not good enough to enable estimates to be made which can be relied on to better than an order of magnitude. The calculation of the probable final level of 'genetic-load' in a population subject to the incursion of radiation induced mutation is even more uncertain. One has at the moment the feeling of over-emphasis on radiation as a cause of genetic change in the population. There could be a number of unknown or only vaguely known physical, biological, chemical and social factors which might be of comparable significance. However, this feeling is obviously not a good basis for recommending the relaxation of vigilance relative to radiation. More knowledge in many fields is the first requirement and co-ordinated researches in human genetics and environmental factors in general are urgently required.

My general worry about the numerical values of I.C.R.P. recommendations (and I must add that for a number of years I was a member of the Commission and must therefore accept some responsibility) is the weakness of the biological and medical foundations coupled with a most impressive numerical façade. The original selection of numbers for the so-called 'tolerance dose' for radiation workers was based largely on the production of blood changes due to whole-body exposure from low-voltage X rays, and we may legitimately wonder whether it is reasonable to use essentially o.3 rad per week for the 'maximum permissible' dose rate in individual organs. It is usually a relatively simple calculation to find the amount of a radioactive material uniformly deposited throughout a given organ to give a mean dose of say, o.3 rad per week, but the actual exposure usually has a complex time pattern and often the fraction of the dose in a given organ is very inadequately known. I have already indicated some of the complexities of micro-dosimetry. The mathematical assumption of exponential or power series expressions for the time-variation of concentration in a given organ or whole body is often an over-simplification and much more complex patterns are in fact followed.

My complaint is that by setting the computers humming and calculating a most impressive and consistent set of numbers (and it is only fair to add useful and comforting numbers) showing the maximum permissible amounts of large numbers of radioactive materials in many organs, we give a false impression of certainty; comforting to administrators but not quite so comfortable to live with as scientists. The calculations give us correctly the concentration of radioactive material which will deliver a given dose; the difficult question arises whether this is the right dose. Perhaps physicists think biology is not their concern; biologists have difficulty with the sums and the medical man has given up arguing though he feels a faint malaise at the sudden consistency of his prospective patients.

It is very difficult to find a better basis for decisions and at least one thing can be said of the numbers suggested by I.C.R.P., namely, that (to my knowledge) they have never led to disaster. So far as I know, it has never been shown that a person has been damaged by occupational irradiation at the levels laid down by the Commission, and this in itself is a great deal. It would be less easy to answer the question as to whether they have ever been unnecessarily restrictive.

I have the impression, too, that when changes of allowed level are to be introduced they are often insufficiently explained and justified to the ordinary user. No change should be made unless absolutely necessary and the precise reasons for any change must now be explicitly stated. There is much to be said for a system of publication of suggested change as a provisional measure followed by a period of discussion of possible objections. This tends to remove the impression of arbitrary decision from above and gives the opportunity to assess 'quantitatively' the advantages and disadvantages of the proposals.

It is instructive to turn to a very different field of hazard and to compare these radiation recommendations with those applicable in the field of chemical toxicology of metals. Again, we meet the same two main classes of problem, the high exposure of a limited number of persons in a particular industry or group of industries, and alternatively possible effects on the population as a whole subjected to very low levels of continued contamination with a resulting build-up of low concentrations of materials in their tissues.

I know of no evidence that tissue concentrations of metals now observed have so far caused disease, but in the concentrations encountered in industry there are, of course, serious toxic effects and local injury in for example respiratory organs. Systemic poisoning may reveal a wide range of symptoms in the central nervous system (lead, manganese), the liver (arsenic) or in bone (beryllium). Some metals may be carcinogenic as, for example, arsenic, chromium, nickel and possibly beryllium. Since inhalation plays such an important part in chemical toxicity it is not surprising that the usual parameter fixed is 'maximum allowable concentration' (M.A.C.) in air. This quantity is defined as 'that average concentration in air that causes no signs or symptoms of illness or physical impairment in all but hypersensitive workers during their working day on a continuing basis, as judged by the most sensitive internationally accepted test'. It is emphasized that constant effort must be made to reduce the concentration to considerably lower levels or 'as far as possible within reasonable limits of cost'.

Let us look at the corresponding radiation definition. 'The permissible dose,' says I.C.R.P., 'for an individual is that dose, accumulated over a long period of time or resulting from a single exposure, that in the light of present knowledge carries a negligible probability of severe somatic or genetic injuries. Furthermore, it is such a dose that any effects that ensue more frequently are limited to those of a minor nature that would not be considered unacceptable by

the exposed individual and by competent medical authori-
ties.' 'The permissible dose,' says I.C.R.P., 'can therefore
be expected to produce effects that could be detected only
by statistical methods applied to large groups'. I expect
that it will have been noted with pleasure that whatever
the computer may say the poor doctor in the end still
decides! It will also have been noted that I.C.R.P. is
more rigorous and more cautious than its chemical counter-
part. I do not know of attempts to set levels for the general
population in the chemical field. Reliance is placed in a
'threshold' philosophy.

Chapter 8

COMPARATIVE RISKS AND ADVANTAGES

During the last year or two there has been increasing interest in the question 'What is a permissible dose'? or, more fundamentally, 'What is a permissible risk; permissible for whom and by whom'? This interest inevitably leads to an attempt to estimate the risks associated with radiation and compare them with others met with in our society.

These and related questions have been admirably discussed by Dr. Pochin,[31] the present chairman of I.C.R.P., who points out that we should not ask what is the safe dose, but rather what is the safety of the dose. He takes the view that the real decision to be made in fixing levels of radiation is the permissible risk under particular circumstances, taking into account the source and need for radiation exposure, the number and ages of the people involved, and whether the exposure occurs in the course of their occupation. In order to obtain a balanced view we must also attempt to estimate quantitatively the benefits that may be associated with any particular procedure involving radiation exposure. Clearly, the risk must in any circumstances be made as low as practicable and continuing effort must be made to keep it low or perhaps bring it even lower, but opinions will differ as to what is practicable.

The question of comparative risks from radiation and other hazards of life has also been ably discussed in a report published by World Health Organization in 1962[32] and in a seminar organized by special agencies of the United Nations in December 1961.[33] Here we can only summarize a very wide range of material.

In the greater part of the world in its relatively undeveloped state, the main health problems are infant mortality, malnutrition and communicable disease. It is hardly necessary to remind readers that in advanced countries degenerative diseases, malignant neoplasms, respiratory diseases and accidents usurp their pride of place. The world's large-scale needs are for good food and water. It has been estimated that each year 500 million people suffer from disabling diseases associated with unsafe water supplies. Apart from more humane considerations, this results in a stupendous loss of man-hours. Because of their own direct needs for water, industry and commerce tend to avoid areas where supplies are inadequate, so that the economic effects of poor water supplies can thus also be extremely serious.

The figures of incidence of major diseases are impressive. Two hundred million people in the world suffer from malaria, 400 million from trachoma, 150 million from bilharziasis. Malaria is estimated to occur among one-third of the world's population and in 1959 to have caused about 1 million deaths. In England and Wales neoplasms in 1959 caused 214, and cardiovascular diseases 535 deaths per 100,000 population.

In the younger age-groups, even in 1955, the man-years estimated to be lost due to deaths of persons between 20 and 29 years of age in motor vehicle accidents in the United States was estimated at over 420,000, about one-third of the corresponding loss from all causes. Sowby[34] has recently collected interesting data on these subjects, expressing risks as death rates per hour per 10^9 population, thus enabling comparisons to be made between various forms of human disease, accident and folly. When we look at the risk of malignant neoplasms in our population we find that in males (with the exception of lung cancer) the neoplasms of concern to 'health physics', that is of a type most commonly attributed to radiation (leukæmia, cancer of skin and bone) are low risks. Cancer of skin and bone have very low rates of incidence and in the past 10 years there has been a tendency for them to drop. Leukæmia accounts for about 2.5 per cent of neoplasms in the male (about 0.5 per cent of all causes of death).

Motor vehicle accidents are an important cause of death in most advanced countries. In Great Britain nearly 7,000 people were killed in road accidents in 1963 and this number steadily increases. Sowby has estimated the death rates per 10^9 occupant-hours for various types of road vehicles and demonstrated the large variation between motor-cyclists (6,600) and public service vehicles (30). Rail travel has a very low risk. If we are thinking of death rate alone the transfer of passengers from roads to trains would provide an excellent safety measure which could save many more lives than any radiation safety measure I could think of. Flying is relatively safe per mile, but not per hour. As Sowby puts it, 'for a journey of a certain distance it is safer to travel by plane than by car, and very much safer by bus or train. But if one wishes to while away an hour, it is much safer to take a sightseeing bus than a sightseeing plane or motor-car'.

When one looks at the occupational hazards there are very large differences of risk between industries. Indeed, the differences are glaringly apparent. Construction engineers and erectors, railway shunters, level crossing men, coal miners, fishermen, have ranges from 675 to 330 expressed as death rate per hour per 10^9 persons, whereas medical practitioners and radiologists (the distinction is the Registrar-General's, not mine!) suffer 60. Disease incidence has fascinating occupational patterns. Why is cancer of the lung high in publicans, barmen, painters and decorators, whereas the incidence among clergy of the Church of England is very low?

There is much less variation of incidence of leukæmia with occupation, but the numbers of cases are small per industry (600 to 800 in various industries in four years). There is no gross increase in the rates of leukæmia in the medical practitioner group but, of course, many are not occupationally exposed to radiation and there is some evidence of higher rates in the radiological groups.

In order to maintain our 'balanced' view we may look at a great variety of other impressive numbers such as those relating to chemical toxicity in world industry; in Germany 3,000 to 4,000 new cases per annum of silicosis in coal miners, in Italy 80,000 people exposed to a real hazard of silicosis. In the last 50 years lead has caused several thousand fatal cases of poisoning. The catalogue can continue indefinitely and I choose at random. We are well aware of recent concern at the increasing pollution of air, food and water. A recent report from the U.S.A. shows that pesticides cause about one death per million population per year. The avenues of ingress are not only the obvious ones. Residues left in clothing by cleaning solvents and moth-proofing solutions, furnace filters and paper used in the kitchen may transmit pesticides to man. Pesticides may accumulate in living tissue with the result that unforeseen irrevocable and undesirable side effects have arisen 'on a sizeable scale'. A famous 'smog' caused the deaths of 4,000 people in London during a seven-day period. Thousands of cases of fatal chronic bronchitis in England per year are thought to be caused by irritating substances in the air. We think of carcinogenesis associated with industrial materials such as complex hydrocarbons, benzidine and beta-naphthylamine, or of chromium, nickel and asbestos; of the possible effects of additives to food; the use of œstrogens in agriculture and, last but not least, the risks associated with smoking.

An interesting table given in summary by Sowby shows a very rough classification of overall risks. They cover a vast range ($1-500,000$ per 10^9 per hour), but certainly radio-logical risks (cancer of skin and bone and leukæmia) fall in the lowest category. It is probable that the present maxi-mum permissible occupational dose (5 rem per year) would not more than treble the low risk of leukæmia. The num-ber of people exposed even to such levels of radiation is very small. It seems that risks less than 10 on Sowby's scale (cancer of skin, bone, leukæmia) cause little social concern (except in the case of leukæmia) and a rough boundary of 100 lies between acceptability and non-acceptability. Among risks over 100 one finds lung cancer, accidents and pneumoconiosis in coal miners, accidents in coal mines and on the roads, cardiovascular diseases and car accidents. Some very high risks are associated with sports (rock climbing and professional boxing). These have all given rise to anxiety. A second criterion seems to be that some very high risks are accepted provided the actual number of deaths is very small as, for example, in such sports as boxing and horse racing.

Comparing these numbers with the low rates of radiation accidents and moderate irradiation risks in the atomic energy industry and even in industry generally, we may reach the comforting conclusion that radiation is numerically at present one of the smaller risks in industrial society. That the number of deaths and injuries reasonably attributable to radiation is very small there can be no doubt; it is indeed difficult to find them at all. The occupational hazards of radiation are a very small fraction of the total industrial hazard, but this does not, of course, absolve us from the necessity to reduce it to a minimum and no one doubts the potential hazards of natural and artificial radioactive substances. I think more effort could be made to express the whole radiation situation numerically. In particular, I can imagine much argument about what is the hidden genetic hazard not applicable to some other risks. It could be zero, but it might not, and this is surely one of the most important points at issue.

However, we have as yet not looked at the positive side of the account. It is doubtless part of the wisdom of the medical profession that it rarely, so far as I know, attempts to assess in the grand manner either the good or the harm it does, and this perhaps accounts for the rather strange silence in a blatant world on the positive contribution to the community of radiation in medical hands. In 1957 it is estimated that 13 million radiological examinations were carried out in the British National Health Service Hospitals. We know fairly accurately the genetic dose delivered in that period. We may make, if we wish, estimates of the numbers of leukæmias so 'caused', but no one ever seems to have calculated how many people lived reasonably happy lives for how much longer as the result of those examinations, how many anxieties were relieved, or how many times they facilitated effective treatment. Quantitative data of this kind are conspicuously lacking. The Adrian Committee[13] modestly referred to the undoubted benefits which are conferred upon the individual and the population by diagnostic and therapeutic radiology. In its interim report it noted that mass miniature radiography in 1957 revealed 17,835 cases of pulmonary tuberculosis. Over 63,000 other abnormalities were detected including 2,363 cases of lung cancer, 12,000 cardiac abnormalities and 9,400 cases of pneumoconiosis.

In the same year about 60,000 patients in this country were treated radiologically for non-malignant conditions. About the same number were treated for malignant disease, the main sites of treatment being lung, breast, cervix and skin, buccal cavity and pharynx. In *Supplements on Cancer* 1952–53 the Registrar-General has given survival rates for five to seven years after the treatment of malignant disease at 14 sites, and it might be interesting to study them and see what effects in patient-years were produced by treatment.

I can imagine the seeker for numerical data also turning to such publications as the *Annual Report on the Results of Treatment in Carcinoma of the Uterus*, collated in 1960 by the International Federation of Gynæcology and Obstetrics,[35] which gives the results from 1945 to 1954 on 97,495 cases of carcinoma of the uterus treated in 23 countries. The whole series of reports concerns 186,591 examined cases of uterine carcinoma. It would be an interesting exercise, again, to try to determine quantitative data for such figures as the increase of useful life and its significance, apportioning between surgery and radiotherapy. The attempt to calculate utility in this way is possibly absurd, but probably no more absurd than many of the other data we have already considered and it might also be a salutary exercise in radio-therapeutic research. We again meet the fundamental difficulty of defining 'health' and expressing it by a statistic. It is easy to give numbers of deaths due to disease, but not for health and its improvement. As Sir Robert Platt[36] remarked last year while discussing antibiotics and tonsillitis in children: 'It is easy to estimate the drug bill. It is quite impossible to estimate even the financial gain of rescuing a few children from invalidism, hospital treatment and deafness'.

Any attempt to balance the utility and risk of radiation must also discuss the social consequences of the release and application in peace-time of atomic energy. I have deliberately excluded from this discussion its war-time significance. How important is this new source of power to health and in what ways might it improve the health of the community? There has, of course, been great enthusiasm, in which I share, followed by some disappointment. The development of atomic power stations has gone ahead reasonably rapidly in this country, but the fossil fuel supplies and stations using them have shown a surprising resilience so that parity of cost has not yet been achieved. In the world at large the impact of atomic power has been slow. If the cost of electric power is reduced this may make little difference to costs in some industries and in many agricultural countries where the population is scattered the very large efficient power stations are not suited to the need.

Suppose, however, we could all have electric power

much more cheaply and easily, how do we estimate the gain to the health of the community? Better goods at the same or reduced price raise the standard of living, but it is difficult to separate the financial advantage of the manufacturer from the material and social advantage to the public, or from the economic gains of the community as a whole.

Economic surveys made under varying conditions and with differing assumptions disagree by orders of magnitude in their estimates of the saving to industry by the use of radioactive isotopes; for example, they vary from 140 million pounds equivalent in the United States to 14 million. In 1957–58 in the United Kingdom it was estimated that the use of radioactive isotopes was saving some £3.5 million per annum[37, 38, 39]. The preliminary report of a survey at present in progress by the International Atomic Energy Agency in which Great Britain is participating, suggests £9 million to £12 million overall saving to industry. The uses are varied from studies of silting of docks and harbours to the design of electric generators, gamma radiography and industrial research, but often most profitable in smaller items. The most widely applied radioisotope technique in industry is the use of nucleonic thickness-gauging devices. The extent of the use of isotopes may be inferred from the fact that in 1963–64 the Radiochemical Centre, Amersham, despatched 49,000 consignments and the sale of radioactive products reached £1,621,000.

The gain to the health of the community by the use of isotopes in medicine is still more difficult to assess. The utilization of iodine 131 in the study of the thyroid, the use of phosphorus 32 therapeutically, cobalt 60 and caesium 137 in powerful external sources replacing X-ray equipment as well as hundreds of labelled compounds are well known and need no description, but how the economic gain due to more rapid diagnosis or treatment and return of patients to productive employment, to say nothing of lower costs of maintaining patients in hospitals can be assessed, I do not know. Economically we can guess, but 'health-wise' what standards do we use? New techniques on the verge of medicine continually add their quota of usefulness. Radio-sterilization in surgical and pharmaceutical industries and the probability of food sterilization on a large scale may affect the health of the community. The Atomic Energy Authority reports that a package irradiation plant containing 320,000 curies is used to capacity by industrial firms to demonstrate the commercial feasibility of gamma radiation as a method of sterilizing medical equipment and pharmaceuticals. The first plants are intended for sterilizing plastic hypodermic syringes and surgical sutures. Sometimes sterilization by gamma irradiation in sealed containers gives a shelf-life of several years compared to a few weeks by traditional methods. The economic gain will have less and less meaning as radioisotope techniques become more fully integrated with other scientific methods and begin to play their part as tools in a broadening region of industry and research.

Atomic power, too, is not just an equal alternative to conventional power. Smoke could disappear with nuclear power and transport of fuels would be negligible. With the rapid urbanization now taking place in industrialized countries it is probable that regulations against air pollution will become so strict that conventional power plants cannot exist within certain city limits. It is surprising, too, that our own measurements of the radioactivity of coal and similar investigations in America show that when the physical and biological properties of the various nuclides are taken into consideration, the conventional fossil fuelled plants discharge at least as large quantities of radioactive materials to the atmosphere as nuclear powered plants of comparable size. Atomic power might provide the solution when we reach the point of being able to look at the operation of reactors with the same confidence as we now look upon gasworks within city limits.

I would suspect, however, that the most important influence of atomic energy and radioactive materials on the health of the world could in the end be via agriculture. Looking at the matter globally, the world's real problems are shortage of food and water, and atomic energy could probably have its greatest effect in reducing loss in production, storage and distribution of food, raising the productivity of land and developing new areas. It could provide cheaper forms of power for pumping water, which for low-lying rivers, swamps and underground sources may be of great importance, or on the other hand desert or semidesert areas may be made suitable for development through the provision of irrigation facilities in many parts of the world. There is great need for power in the forestry industry. About half the world's harvest of wood is now used as fuel and atomic power might allow much needed reconstruction of adequate forest cover. We have already spoken of the use of radiation in food sterilization, although there are many problems here, including the possible production of deleterious substances in the foodstuffs themselves. The destruction of insects in stored foodstuffs such as grain, cereal products and dried fruit, appears to be a particularly promising application of radiation. The present position seems to be that the technical and commercial feasibility is not yet well established. In a slightly different field there is room for the development of nuclear power units of a size and nature suitable for installation in ships as 'mother' or 'factory' vessels in fishing and whaling industries.

Again, one can imagine important applications of radiation in the breeding of improved varieties of plants and animals. The use of new mutations produced by radiation, new strains of barley, wheat and oats, soya beans, flax and many others could be extremely important and at the same time the control of insect pests, as for example the screw worm by sterilization of the male flies, shows what could be accomplished. We are aware of the dangers of ecological interference, but this single action has practically eliminated a pest which was estimated to do 20 million dollars worth of damage annually in the south-east of the United States.

Radioactive isotopes thus have an extremely wide range of applications in research in agriculture, fisheries, forestry and human nutrition and may well aid in the development of better methods of producing and utilizing food and agricultural products. With the aid of isotopes an investigator can sometimes achieve results not obtainable in any other way and he can do so with greater certainty and more cheaply.

In the long run the contribution that radioactive isotopes and radiation can make to increased food production and to the more effective utilization of agricultural products may turn out to be as important as the more obvious and more spectacular impact that atomic energy makes as a source of industrial power. The improved standard of health may then encourage still more efficient food production and thus assist in the world's overpopulation problem.

I see no way of attaining these goals without some radiation risk. Ionizing radiation is the outcome, at present the inseparable companion to the release of atomic energy, for it is the means whereby the disturbed and fractured atom returns to relative stability and calm. 'Radiation and health' is one facet of the newly-available form of energy in human life, but the relation between radiation and electric-power production could change rapidly if more direct methods of attaining nuclear energy were discovered. There is at the present time intense research into methods of raising the temperature of gases to millions or even hundreds of millions of degrees centigrade for short intervals of time, thus enabling nuclear reactions to proceed and liberate energy. Of course, no material walls can contain such high temperature 'plasma' which has to be held by intense magnetic fields which unfortunately prove very unstable, allowing the plasma to escape from its magnetic cage. Exploratory work on a modest scale is also in progress on methods for the direct conversion of heat to electrical energy.

Should, however, these fusion processes replace the present fission techniques of liberating energy the radiation hazards due to the production of radioactive materials in the present reactors would largely disappear. I do not know of any detailed forecasts of hazards in the vicinity of the possible new fusion establishments, but there would probably be very intense X-ray beams and neutron atmospheres, but these are local problems. Some at least of the hazards would decrease, though radioactive isotopes are now so useful that we would still have to make them deliberately, but probably in much smaller quantities.

SUMMARY

We commenced this survey with a list compiled a few years ago of environmental factors then thought of social importance. Radiation was not included, but has recently attracted so much attention as almost to monopolize the centre of the stage. Always socially the Ugly Sister of handsome Atomic Energy, Radiation's entry was greeted with suspicion from the beginning and few noticed that she had previously been standing modestly in the wings.

Humanity's first introduction to nuclear power was the explosion of an atomic bomb. It is exceedingly difficult for most people to keep the productive uses of atomic energy clearly separated in their minds from its destructive possibilities. Ionizing radiations were first used in medicine for the diagnosis and treatment of some of the most alarming diseases such as tuberculosis or cancer. All these circumstances contribute to making the concept of atomic energy unduly frightening.[40]

Moreover, the thought that so gigantic a force can be produced by the dissolution of so exceedingly small a quantity of matter and that radiations cannot be seen, heard, smelled, tasted or felt, yet may produce profound effects on those exposed and their offspring must inevitably provoke irrational and, maybe, some reasonable fears. Atomic energy is increasing the speed of human social and technical development and an unstable emotional state and unsatisfactory human relationships tend to increase with social disorganization. I do not consider here the political and military questions involved, though atomic energy is often seen as an important bastion of economic power, and this in its turn is one of the mainsprings of political power

I wonder if it is too fanciful to recall also that men have always experienced intense anxiety at the moment of increase of knowledge and power, an anxiety universally reflected in myth and legend. Increase of knowledge and the punishment coupled with it are vividly drawn in the story of the Garden of Eden. Prometheus in stealing fire, the prerogative of the gods, came to understand this prerogative but appropriated it for the use of men and was terribly punished. Pandora freed Spites she could not control, but since her action was accidental, and some say innocent, she was left in the end with Delusive Hope.

Many circumstances led to a fear of radiation which it is hard to combat. Also, at a far less exalted literary level here was the press headline writer's dream—horror, mass destruction, invisible death rays, ignorance, mystery, cancer, sex—it had everything.

In an effort to attain some reasonable balance of emphasis we have examined some of the other risks to which mankind is exposed and some of the contributions which radiation and atomic power have made or might make in our society. We have seen that numerically the risks of radiation effects on the community are minimal compared to the impact of the world's existing major diseases or social and nutritional needs. I sought in some measure to balance numerically 'good' and 'evil', 'utility' and 'risk', and as time went on I found the attempt a delusion. At first much attracted by the 'comparative-risk' philosophy, I now doubt if it will carry us very far. The allowable risk, the allowed extent of the use of radiation by our society, cannot depend on such numbers. The allowable risk to a radiation worker cannot depend on whether 50 or 1,000 men die in a far-off country of silicosis or whether thousands are poisoned by lead. The numerical data serve to illuminate starkly the absurdities of the relative emphasis placed on radiation hazards relative to others, but that is all. It is still our duty to preserve the gain and minimize the risk. Besides, I had an awful vision of a succession of monographs such as this in a contest for public favour. I imagined a group of the building industry glossing their high accident rate with glowing terms which set out 'the contribution to health and well-being of the community through good housing for the people'. I am almost inspired to do the farmer's spiritual accountancy myself in terms of 'good and whole-some food' did I not know that they could do it better for themselves. In the end we must look at the numbers and make the most sensible decision we can, crying with John Donne[41] as he ends his satirical poem:

'There's nothing simply good, nor ill alone,
Of every quality comparison
The only measure is, and judge, opinion.'

There are important questions here of the relativity of fundamental human needs. If mankind really desired atomic energy and radiation on a great scale I fear it would pay for them without noticing, just as it pays for other desires in the holocaust on the roads. Rock Carling years ago warned us that the question might be settled by business men, not men of science, and exhorted the experts to raise their voices and speak from sure ground.

Not that I doubt that there is much useful work to be done in attempting to collect quantitative social data; the results of radiation therapy and diagnosis, the comparison of varying industrial standards and criteria of behaviour, the contradictory definitions of the same quantity (for example of 'a radioactive substance') in varied contexts, such things might well exercise our attention but are technical matters at a different level of decision. Before a new restrictive level is imposed, before a new category of controlled persons is defined, let us sit down in a quantitative mood and ask how many instances of what diseases or disabilities can the proposed measure reasonably be expected to prevent or mitigate. Alternatively, what positive advantages may be expected to accrue from its application. What advantages, hardships, restriction or social chaos will it impose, all expressed in hard numbers? Dare we ask ourselves frankly what would be the quantitative results of either tightening or relaxing all the fundamental maximum permissible levels for the various population groups by, say, a factor of three, or even ten.

I have myself sat spellbound as well-meaning administrators proposed to set in motion measures which would have caused untold social confusion and alarm, because a single measurement of concentration of a radioactive material approached a level set for years of continuous consumption.

It is always easy to think of reasons for additional safeguards or for relaxed standards, and the larger the committee the greater the chance that someone will. 'In the multitude of counsellors there is safety' (Prov. xi, 14)—for the 'counsellors' too.

The atomic industry has from its start been so safety-minded that there is reason to hope that when more experience has been gained the trend may be towards softening and simplification of present practices and measures. This would contrast with customary development in industry where restrictive measures are normally only laid down when pollution has reached such levels that the inconvenience and risks are clearly demonstrable. The simplification is important. I have been involved with these matters for many years, but have great sympathy with those who find the present plethora of texts controlling radiation unnecessarily complex and confusing. As I have explained, the fundamental numbers mostly stem from one source, yet each Ministry, each Department, each Board, finds it necessary to set up its own committee structure and to add its own gloss on the text. In so far as this is educational in the organization concerned and brings greater safety to those involved such action is excellent, but it often wastes and diverts valuable administrative and scientific manpower. It also produces frustration and inhibition in daily implementation. The utmost effort should be made to attain simplicity and consistency. Let us face the fact that radiation is an omnipresent feature of our society and that the circumstances in which it may be encountered are so multitudinous that to attempt to define them all and to specify appropriate behaviour for each is ridiculous.

I hope I shall not be misunderstood. Radiation carries its own subtle brand of danger which must be defined and controlled. I am not advocating relaxation of standards, but a new appraisal of the limits of our ignorance, further attempts to reduce that ignorance, and an effort to simplify existing and future control. We remember, too, depressing though the idea may be to scientists, that control of hazard will in some measure be arbitrary and based in ignorance. I know of no instance in which it has been dependent upon detailed knowledge and understanding of cellular or sub-cellular mechanisms.

As we look at the whole pattern one or two themes continually recur; we always see leukæmia, genetics, diagnostic radiology. Why the emphasis on these? Leukæmia is according to our numerical philosophy a triviality. I think its prominence stems from several circumstances. First, because it seems to be one of the most sensitive indicators of population irradiation—a warning light whose intermittent flashing catches our attention. It is a rising risk and associated with young children and an emotional appeal of a very fundamental kind; it is largely still incurable. To scientists it has the appeal of a field from which there is hope that fundamental information may be gleaned to enlarge and perhaps change our views of malignant disease in general.

There is no need to set forth reasons for the prominence of the genetic problem. It is obvious. Technically it happens that radiation is a powerful and subtle tool for bringing about changes in hereditary material. There may be many others less obvious and less susceptible of quantitative appraisal yet equally cogent in determining the future structure of the race. Radiation suffers one suspects from being at the moment too conspicuous among the known effective agents of genetic ills. I cannot believe that the radiation levels of the present day constitute a major human genetic hazard.

I have deliberately laid emphasis upon the study of natural ionizing radiation to which the whole surface of the earth in varying degrees is and has been subject, as well as upon the universal presence of natural radioactive substances in our own bodies and in our environment. This emphasis arises from no naïve intuition that if a thing is 'natural' it 'does you good' or at least no harm. Neither is it merely for the psychological comfort of knowing that irradiation of the human race did not begin with the atom bomb, though this was important. Its importance lies rather in the demonstration that levels of irradiation exist at which no obvious and gross deleterious effects are produced, indeed levels at which rather disappointingly even our careful searches have so far demonstrated no effects whatever. Maybe we have not looked very carefully or intelligently so far. We certainly must continue searching if for no other reason than to further the study of the significance of radiation in evolution. The knowledge that evolution has taken place in a radiation field of even higher intensity than now existing may well argue that mechanisms of repair and deletion may exist of which we are unaware. Natural selection must, one would think, evoke mechanisms for the control of its own means of action and the means of controlling mutation rate must be an important part of evolutionary mechanism.

Diagnostic radiology I have already to some extent defended. Here is social gain of importance and the need is for responsible decision and technical competence in its use and daily control. It is too valuable a tool of modern medicine to be used carelessly or discarded lightly.

In all, I am still a long-term optimist. I have no doubt, provided we avoid nuclear war, that the release of atomic energy and atomic radiation will prove one of humanity's greatest and most rewarding adventures. The gain will be worth the risks.

* * * *

To hold a Rock Carling Fellowship is a high honour, particularly gratifying to one like myself privileged to have known Sir Ernest as an intimate friend. I am the more deeply grateful to the Nuffield Provincial Hospitals Trust for the opportunity to attempt a tribute to him.

It is a measure of the breadth of Rock Carling's interests that a physicist should be called upon so early in the series to attempt a survey of one of them. Radiation and its control was the stimulus for his 'second professional life' from which he obtained so much satisfaction and which perhaps displayed at their fullest his administrative ability and maturity of judgement. His width of interests and detailed knowledge of a range of sciences were important at a critical moment in the history of the utilization of radiation, but, at a more profound level, he knew well the arts which suffuse scientific progress with human understanding and so transform its significance.

References

REFERENCES

1. Charles, Sir John, *The Social Context of Medicine*, The Nuffield Provincial Hospitals Trust, 1962.
2. Brockington, C. Fraser, *World Health*, Penguin Books, 1958.
3. Carling, Sir E. Rock, *Peaceful Uses of Atomic Energy*, Vol. XI, p. 76, Proceedings of the International Conference, Geneva, August 1955.
4. *The Radium Commission. A Short History of its Origin and Work*, 1929–48, H.M. Stationery Office, London, 1951.
5. *The Hazards to Man of Nuclear and Allied Radiations*, Medical Research Council, H.M. Stationery Office, London, 1956 (Cmd. 9780).
6. *The Hazards to Man of Nuclear and Allied Radiations*, A Second Report to the Medical Research Council, H.M. Stationery Office, London, 1960 (Cmnd. 1225).
7. *Report of the United Nations Scientific Committee on the Effects of Atomic Radiation*, United Nations, New York, 1962.
8. *Recommendations of the International Commission on Radiological Protection*, Pergamon Press, London:
   (a) Report of Main Commission, 1959.
   (b) Amended Recommendations, 1964.
   (c) Report of Committee II, *Permissible Dose for Internal Radiation*, 1959.
   (d) Report of Committee III, *Protection against X-rays up to energies of 3 meV and Beta and Gamma Rays from Sealed Sources*, 1960.
   (e) Report of Committee IV, *Protection against Electro-*

magnetic Radiation above 3 meV and Electrons, Neutrons and Protons, 1964.

9. *World Health Organization Chronicle*, Vol. 15, p. 445, December 1961.

10. *The Effects of Nuclear Weapons*, Ed. S. Glasstone, Washungton, D.C., 1962.

11. Loutit, J. F., *Irradiation of Mice and Men*, University of Chicago Press, 1962.

12. Court-Brown, W. M. and Doll, R., *Leukæmia and Aplastic Anæmia in Patients Irradiated for Ankylosing Spondylitis*, Medical Research Council Special Report Series No. 295, H.M. Stationery Office, London, 1957.

13. *Radiological Hazards to Patients*, Second Report, H.M. Stationery Office, London, 1960.

14. Wallace, B. and Dobzhansky, Th., *Radiation, Genes, and Man*, Holt, Rinehart & Winston Inc., New York, 1963.

15. *Nuclear Radiation in Geophysics*, Ed. H. Israel and A. Krebs, Springer-Verlag, Berlin, 1962.

16. Folsom, T. R. and Harley, J. H., *Comparison of Some Natural Radiations Received by Selected Organisms*, Chap. 2 in The Effects of Atomic Radiation on Oceanography and Fisheries, p. 28, National Academy of Sciences, National Research Council Publication 551, Washington, D.C., 1957.

17. Bugher, J. C. and Mead, P. A., *Peaceful Uses of Atomic Energy*, Vol. 23, p. 165, Proceedings of the Second International Conference, Geneva, September 1958.

18. *Effect of Radiation on Human Heredity*, World Health Organization Technical Report Series No. 166, Geneva, 1959.

19. Krebs, A. and Stewart, N. G., *Biological Aspects, Nuclear Radiation in Geophysics*, p. 241, Springer-Verlag, Berlin, 1962.

20. Agricultural Research Council Radiobiological Laboratory Reports, 1959–63 (ARCRL 1–8), H.M. Stationery Office, London.

21. *Radioactive Materials in Food and Agriculture*, Food and Agricultural Organization of the United Nations, Rome, 1960.

22. *Dietary Levels of Strontium 90 and Caesium 137*, Food and Agricultural Organization of the United Nations, Rome, 1962.

23. *United Kingdom Atomic Energy Authority, Tenth Annual Report*, 1963–64, H.M. Stationery Office, London.

24. *The Control of Radioactive Wastes*, H.M. Stationery Office, London, 1960 (Cmnd. 884).

25. MacMahon, B., *Prenatal X-ray Exposure and Childhood Cancer*, J. Nat. Cancer Inst., Vol. 28, 1173, 1962.

26. Eddington, A. S., *The Nature of the Physical World*, p. 301, Cambridge University Press, 1928.

27. *Background Material for the Development of Radiation Protection*, Federal Radiation Council, Washington, D.C., May 1960 and September 1961.

28. *International Recommendations for X-ray and Radium Protection*, Chicago, September 1937.

29. Wintz, H. and Rump, W., *Protective Measures against Dangers resulting from the Use of Radium, Roentgen and Ultra-violet Rays*, League of Nations Health Organization, Geneva, 1931.

30. Recommendations of the International Commission on

Radiological Protection, London, July 1950, Brit. J. Radiol., Vol. 24, January 1951.

31. Pochin, E. E., *What is a Permissible Dose?* Health Physics, Vol. 9, p. 1091, 1963.

32. *Radiation Hazards in Perspective*, World Health Organization Technical Report Series, No. 248, Geneva, 1962.

33. *Agricultural and Public Health Aspects of Radioactive Contamination in Normal and Emergency Situations*, Food and Agricultural Organization of the United Nations, Rome, 1962.

34. Sowby, F. D., *Radiation and Other Risks*, Health Physics, in press.

35. *Annual Report on the Results of Treatment in Carcinoma of the Uterus*, International Federation of Gynecology and Obstetrics, Ed. H. L. Kottmeier, Stockholm, 1961.

36. Platt, Sir Robert, *Doctor and Patient*, The Nuffield Provincial Hospitals Trust, 1963.

37. Putman, J. L., *Isotopes*, Penguin Books, 1961.

38. Putman, J. L., *Economic Aspects of the Technical Application of Radioisotopes*, Atom, No. 81, p. 213, July 1963.

39. Stuart, D. F. O. and Birch, F., *Survey on the Use of Radioisotopes in British Industry and Industrial Research*, Atom, No. 94, p. 176, August 1964.

40. *Mental Health Aspects of the Peaceful Uses of Atomic Energy*, World Health Organization Technical Report Series No. 151, Geneva, 1958.

41. Donne, John, *The Progress of the Soul*, Poêma Satyricon (1601), J. M. Dent & Sons, p. 244, 1931.

For Product Safety Concerns and Information please contact our EU
representative GPSR@taylorandfrancis.com
Taylor & Francis Verlag GmbH, Kaufingerstraße 24, 80331 München, Germany